Epilepsy During the Lifespan - Beyond the Diagnosis and New Perspectives

Edited by Marco Carotenuto

Published in London, United Kingdom

Epilepsy During the Lifespan - Beyond the Diagnosis and New Perspectives
http://dx.doi.org/10.5772/intechopen.110950
Edited by Marco Carotenuto

Contributors
Bita Shalbafan, Thendo Gertie Makhado, Lufuno Makhado, Congfu Huang, Defeng Cai, Izumi Kuramochi, Takayuki Iwayama, Sakie Shimotsu, Sylvia Tochukwu Echendu, Esther N. Umeadi, Njideka C. Uchefuna, Wilson C. Igwe, Amalachukwu O. Odita, Ngozi N. Joe-Ikechebelu, Izunna S. Okwelogu, Chinonye V. Iloanya, Pavel Vlasov, Aleksander Sobieszek, Isabella D'Andrea-Meira, Marco Carotenuto, Luigi Vetri, Carola Costanza, Margherita Siciliano, Francesco Precenzano, Beatrice Gallai

First published in London, United Kingdom, 2024 by IntechOpen
IntechOpen is the global imprint of INTECHOPEN LIMITED, registered in England and Wales, registration number: 11086078, 5 Princes Gate Court, London, SW7 2QJ, United Kingdom

British Library Cataloguing-in-Publication Data
A catalogue record for this book is available from the British Library

Additional hard and PDF copies can be obtained from orders@intechopen.com

Epilepsy During the Lifespan - Beyond the Diagnosis and New Perspectives
Edited by Marco Carotenuto
p. cm.
Print ISBN 978-1-83769-126-5
Online ISBN 978-1-83769-127-2
eBook (PDF) ISBN 978-1-83769-128-9

For EU product safety concerns:
IN TECH d.o.o., Prolaz Marije Krucifikse Kozulić 3, 51000 Rijeka, Croatia,
info@intechopen.com or visit our website at intechopen.com.

Meet the editor

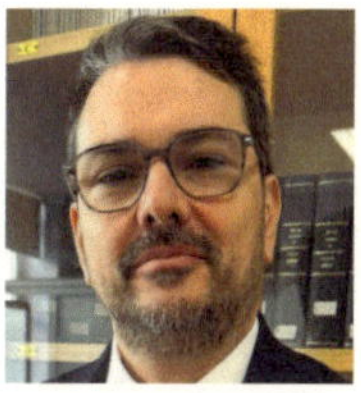

Professor Marco Carotenuto obtained a master's degree in medicine and surgery at the University of Campania "Luigi Vanvitelli," Italy, in 2000. He became a specialist in child neuropsychiatry in 2005 after a long period of training in the United Kingdom. He also obtained a Ph.D. in Behavioral Sciences and Learning Disorders in 2008. In 2018, after further training at prestigious Italian research centers to delve deeper into diagnostic, therapeutic, and rehabilitative issues in developmental age, Dr. Carotenuto became Professor of Child Neuropsychiatry and Director of the Child Neuropsychiatry Unit at the University of Campania "Luigi Vanvitelli." Since 2022, he has been the president of the National Commission for Neurotherapy and Psychomotor Therapy in Developmental Age (TNPEE). Since 2022, he has been Director of the School of Specialization in Child Neuropsychiatry, University of Campania "Luigi Vanvitelli." Dr. Carotenuto has authored more than 200 scientific journal articles. His main areas of research interest include the diagnostic evaluation and therapeutic management of neurodevelopmental disorders with particular attention to childhood autism, sleep disorders, pediatric headaches and epilepsies, and neurocognitive and behavioral rehabilitation in children.

Contents

Preface

Epilepsy is the most frequent neurological pathology in the world and affects individuals of all ages with important effects on neurodevelopment and cognitive and behavioral skills. Despite increasing prevalence and knowledge of the disease, epilepsy is still strongly burdened by social stigma. Treating epileptic pathology is possible thanks to the numerous and various therapeutic techniques now available, many of which do not involve the use of drugs.

The disease affects about 65 million people globally, 80% of whom live in developing countries. The management of epilepsy generally involves antiseizure drugs or surgery for those patients who are candidates. There are also numerous other therapeutic options to support drug therapy such as a ketogenic diet or stimulation of the vagus nerve, in addition to neuromodulation techniques.

Epilepsy has always been cloaked by a mysterious aura. Since ancient times, cultures and civilizations have attempted to understand why a person may appear normal and then suddenly present with intense and uncontrollable convulsions. The first hypothesis indicated a spiritual cause.

Among the oldest texts is one dating back to about 2000 BC written by a Mesopotamian. It describes a patient who has wide eyes and hands, tense feet, and a lack of consciousness. The text attributes the symptoms to the "hand of sin." In 1790 BC, the Hammurabi code listed a "return clause" for slaves who were purchased and subsequently found to experience epileptic crises. The clause was presumably written due to the fear about the cause of the disease. About 700 years after the Hammurabi code was decreed, a Babylonian text outlined a spiritual solution for epileptic patients said to be possessed by evil spirits.

The modern opinion that the etiology of epilepsy is physiological and not divine has its roots largely in the studies of Hippocrates of Kos of 400 BC, who argues that the etiology of epilepsy is precisely similar to that of any other disease, that is, based on physiological principles. This debate between divine and physiological causes would continue for another 2000 years.

Epilepsy is not curable but can be commonly controlled with modern anticonvulsants that prevent convulsions or reduce their intensity. However, more than 30% of people with epilepsy have uncontrolled convulsions even with the best drugs available. Throughout history, epilepsy was viewed with amazement, and uncontrollable convulsions were often attributed to the influence of spirits. It is thought that people in the Stone Age drilled into the skull to dissipate demons. In ancient Greek Hippocratic thought, convulsions were sometimes interpreted as a sign of a person possessing prophetic skills. Early Christian and medieval belief was that epilepsy was a punishment from God, and in early modern times epilepsy was viewed according to the concepts of humoral pathology as a sort of imbalance among the four bodily fluids or humors: blood, phlegm, black bile, and yellow bile.

The first synthetic anticonvulsant, paraldehyde, was introduced in 1882. Subsequently, phenobarbital became the main drug prescribed for epilepsy, followed in 1938 by Difenilhidantoina (Dilantin, phenytoin). Before these drugs, people worldwide depended mainly on plants to treat epileptic convulsions.

Since epilepsy is a disease characterized by sudden and mysterious symptoms, it is not surprising that people have been looking to understand its cause since it was first encountered. The initial attempts to surgically treat epilepsy trace their roots back to Greek, Roman, Egyptian, and South American cultures. Despite the lack of scientific etiology for epilepsy, it was thought that these primitive procedures, which more commonly consisted of drilling, freed the demons that caused the disease. These first surgical concepts are captured in various works of art that span many centuries; the oldest of these artistic references to epilepsy surgery dates back to the late twelfth century.

Recent history shows that public opinion on epilepsy continues to evolve. The second half of the twentieth century, in particular, saw many changes in the treatment by the public of those who have epilepsy. Starting in the 1970s, the United Kingdom began to allow epileptic patients to marry and the United States began to allow them to go to public places such as restaurants and movie theaters. In addition, according to a Gallup survey of Americans from 1949 to 1979, the percentage of the public who said no to the belief that epilepsy is madness has increased from 59% to 92%. The percentage of the public that would allow their children to play with other children with epilepsy had increased from 57% to 89%.

Modern medicine fixes a more physiological logic at the origin of the disease, but there remain critical questions about its mechanism and the most appropriate treatment strategies. This text was born with the idea of providing innovative contributions to epilepsy. Written by scholars on epilepsy worldwide, this book will help readers find new answers to ancient doubts about epilepsy.

Marco Carotenuto
Department of Mental and Physical Health and Preventive Medicine,
University of Campania "Luigi Vanvitelli",
Caserta, Italy

Section 1

New and Old Perspectives on Epilepsy

Chapter 1

Cellular and EEG Patterns of the Reorganization of Cortical Activity in Animal Experimental Models of Epilepsy (in Cats)

Aleksander Sobieszek

Abstract

The aim of this chapter is to present the results of experiments performed in attempt of receiving precise information concerning compositions of the patterns of functional states of the structures of cerebral neocortex, reflected in distributions of intracortical electrical fields including patterns reflecting cellular activity. The data were received in conditions of wakefulness and sleep in cats with permanently implanted cortical electrodes—without necessity of using any pharmacological treatment or in conditions of pharmacological alterations of the functional state of cortical tissue—qualified as ionic (IME) and penicillin (PME) models of epilepsy.

Keywords: HFOs—High frequency oscillations, IcEEG—intracortical electroencephalogram, IME—Ionic model of epilepsy, PME—Penicillin model of epilepsy, GSSM—Gyrus suprasylvian medialis, GSP—Gyrus sigmoideus posterior, FFT—Fast Fourier transfer, HPF—High pass filter, LPF—Low pass filter, NF—Notch filter

1. Introduction

The intention of this research was to gather informations that provide an explanation for various findings. Among others, such as the occurrence of phenomena like ripples and high frequency oscillations (HFOs) in EEG records. These oscillations are widely recognized and accepted as biomarkers indicating the reorganization of cortical activity in epilepsy (For example, see [1–3]). The study was performed in a group of cats with permanently implanted cortical electrodes and, in addition, with implanted subdural cannulae enabling transfer of artificial cerebrospinal fluid with increased concentration of potassium ions in arachnoid space and/or application of appropriate pharmacological substances: IME and PME—experimental models of epilepsy (For example, see [4]). In three cats, intracortical electroencephalogram (IcEEG) was recorded using multicontact concentric electrode: 16 contacts about 40 micrometers each with distance between contacts of 200 micrometers. The experiments were performed with respect to the animals participating in this research, in conditions of quiet wakefulness and sleep. Effects of subdural or intraperitoneal application of penicillin were studied in conditions of general anesthesia, after application of pentobarbital in case of probability of appearance of the clinical epileptic seizures. The first information concerning results of this study was presented during 17th European Congress of Clinical Neurophysiology, Warszawa, 2019 [5].

2. Methods

Figure 1 illustrates the size of the semi-microelectrode in relation to the fragment of cerebral cortex (Nissl stain), localization of implanted electrodes illustrated on the map of cat's brain, and examples of the patterns of cellular discharges. The multi-channel electrode was implanted in the median suprasylvian gyrus (GSSM – gyrus suprasylvianus medialis): number 1 on the map. This is the region of association cortex. Number 2 indicates localization of the second source of information, which is important in this case during evaluation of the functional state of the brain: transcortical macroelectrode (surface electrode versus deep electrode—distance about 3 mm across the cortex)—placed in the somatosensory cortex, close to the motor cortex (GSP – posterior sigmoid gyrus).

The recording of the brain electrical activity in the animals was performed while they were placed in a screened cage. This setup aimed to avoid any alteration of the IcEEG signal caused by electromagnetic fields. The amplifier with a sampling rate of 4 kHz was utilized during the recording process. IcEEG patterns and results of their frequency analysis were presented using equipment offered by ELMIKO—producer of the EEG recording systems.

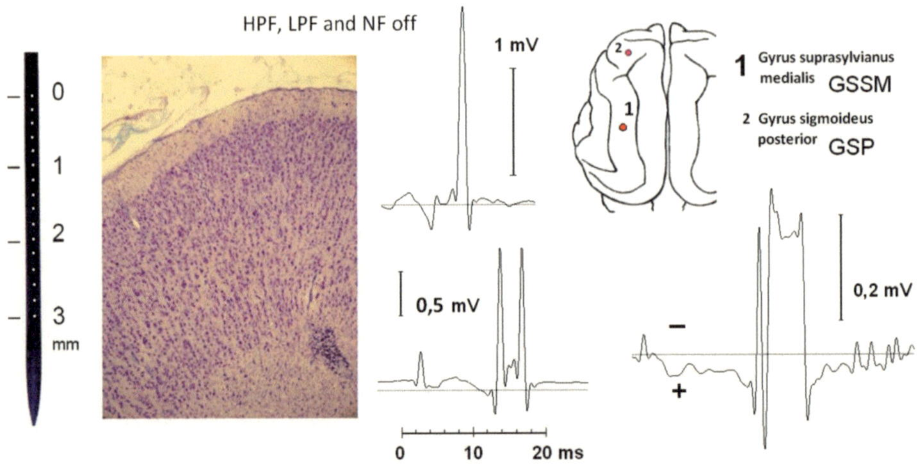

Figure 1.
Illustration of the recording electrode, patterns of cellular discharges and cortical localizations of the implanted electrodes used in this study for evaluation of the functional states of the cerebral cortex. Full description in text.

3. Results

Figure 2(A, B) illustrates the same fragment of IcEEG record: before (**Figure 2A**) and after modification of the EEG pattern (**Figure 2B**) by using different filters: high pass filter (HPF), low pass filter (LPF) and notch filter (NF). This is the fragment of EEG recorded about half a year after implantation of electrodes and on early stage of subdural transfer of artificial cerebrospinal fluid with increased concentration of potassium ions (IME).

Figure 2A illustrates pattern of cortical activity in sleepy animal, presented without using any filtering of the IcEEG record. These are unipolar derivations, with respect to ground. During the experiment, there were instances of scattered spikes within the cortex. These spikes occurred in various locations and sometimes traveled between different layers. The spikes were most frequently observed in cortical layers L3 and L4, specifically in derivations at depths of 0.6 and 0.8 mm. The results of frequency analysis (FFT with analytical window 256 ms) of the EEG fragment

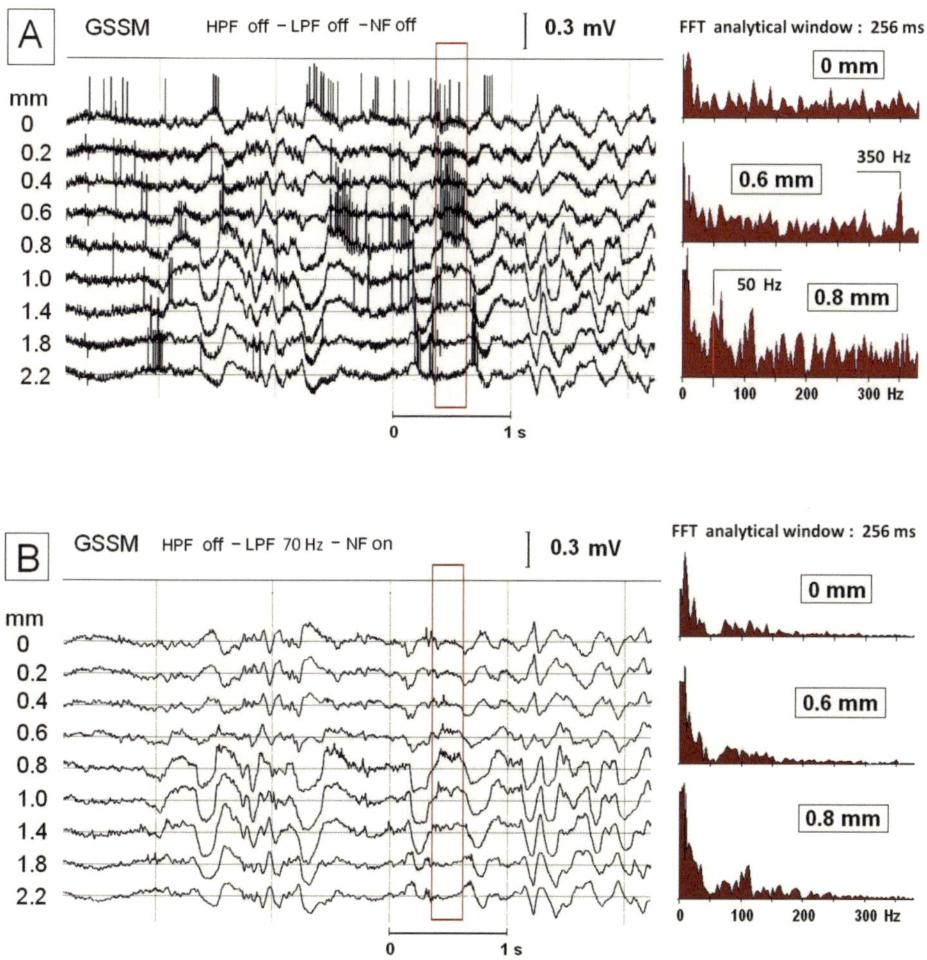

Figure 2.
(A, B). Patterns of the same fragment of IcEEG record: (A) - recorded with all filters switched off, and (B) - presented after filtering using low pass filter (LPF) 70 Hz and notch filter (NF) 50 Hz. Results of frequency analysis (FFT) of selected derivations refer to the IEEG fragment s of 256 ms duration, indictated on the records.

indicated on the IcEEG record illustrate increased activity within the frequency range of 50–60 Hz and 100–120 Hz in derivation from the depth of 0.8 mm and, surprisingly, at about 350 Hz in the derivation at the level of 0.6 mm. This type of information would be unavailable during visual evaluation of this EEG record.

Figure 2B, illustrates effects of using switched on filters: LPF 70 Hz and NF. It confirms appearance of the pattern of Slow Wave Sleep (SWS) during EEG recording with low amplitude ripples in localizations of previously appearing multiple discharges or lack of any signs reflecting existence of the cellular discharges. In **Figure 2B**, due to usage of NF there is a gap in the frequency spectrum around 50 Hz.

Figure 3A, B illustrates similar pattern of widespread, frequent intracortical cellular discharges recorded in the same experiment as illustrated in **Figure 2(A,B)**. This pattern may give impression of existence of the cellular paroxysmal activity. Frequency spectrum of the IcEEG fragment, as shown in **Figure 3A**, illustrates the

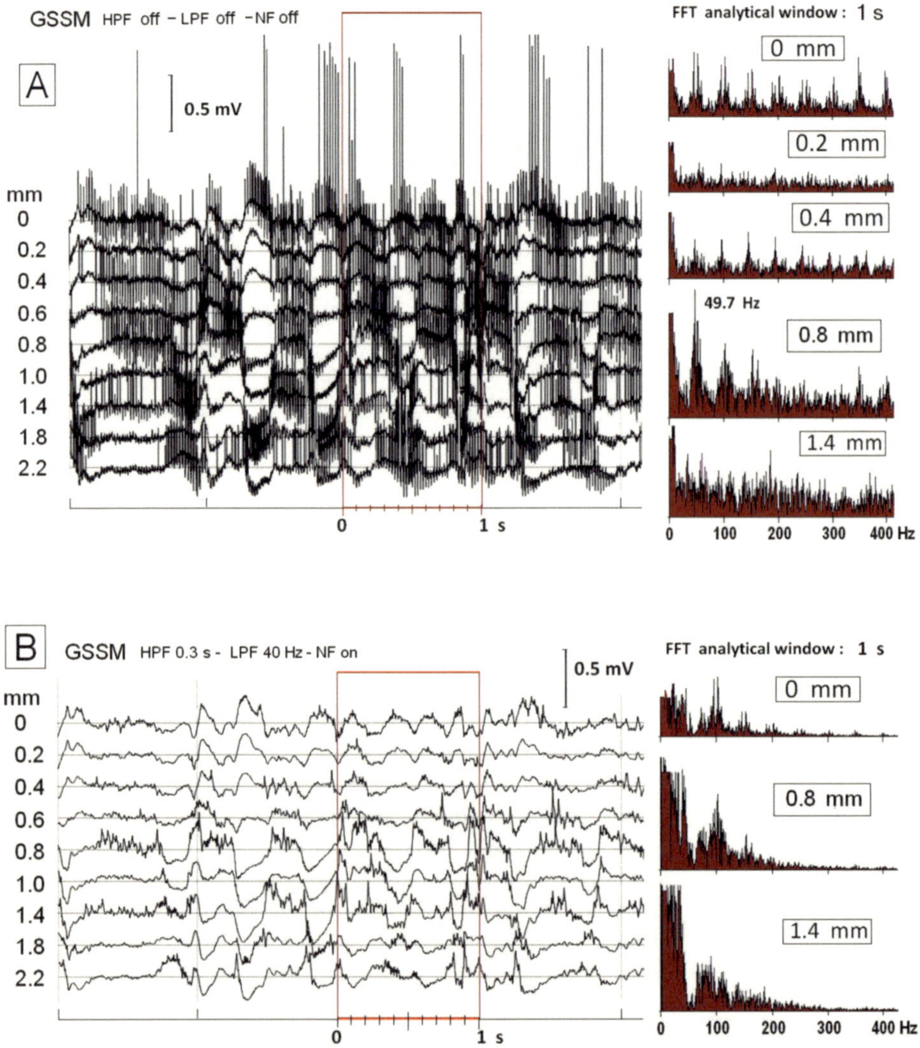

Figure 3.
(A, B). Pattern of IcEEG with greatly intensified appearance of the cellular discharges.

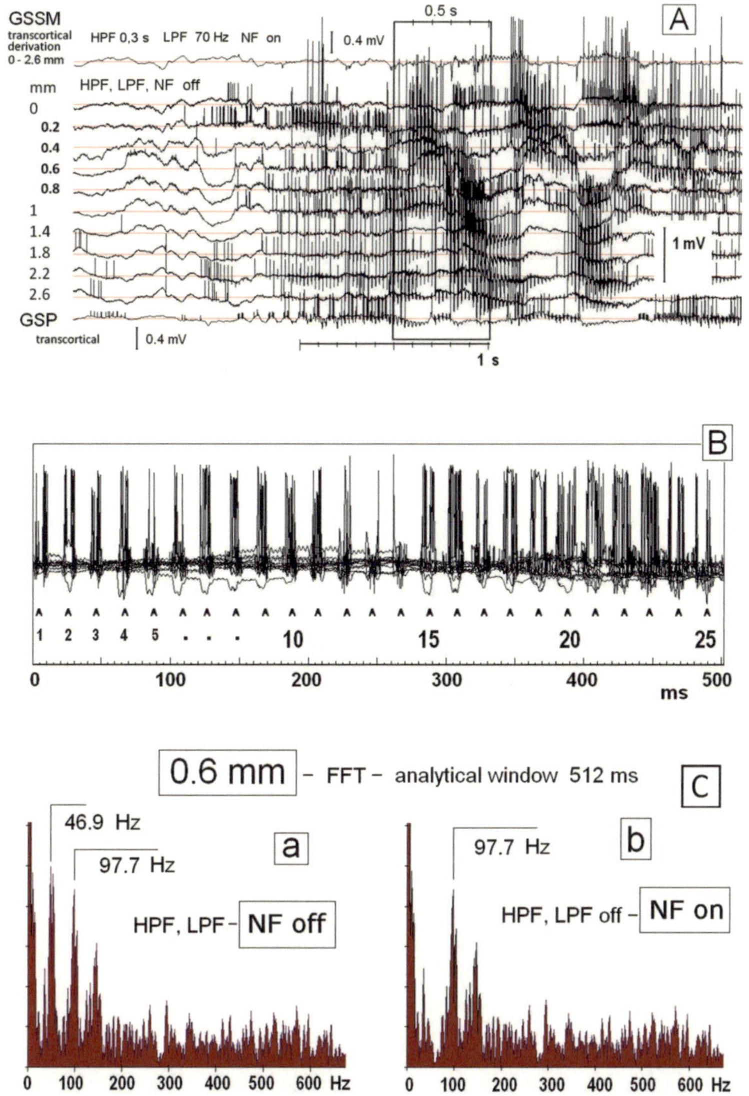

Figure 4.
(A, B, C). Results of visual evaluation of the organization of activity of the cortical generators of the cellular dischages: (A) - IcEEG record with indicated selected fragment illustrating great intensity of spreading cellular dischages (analytical window of 512 ms duration). (B) - after superimposition of all records from the GSSM presented in analytical window - existence of the pattern of rhythmical appearance of the groups of discharges. (C) - results of frequency analysis of the EEG record (in the window) from the depth of 0.6 mm.

existence of great rhythmicity of cellular discharges. There is a prominent peak around 50 Hz, especially evident at the depth of 0.8 mm (49.7 Hz). This indicates a strong rhythmic pattern in the cellular activity within that frequency range.

Figure 3B clearly indicates that the discharges were superimposed on IcEEG patterns of slow wave sleep (SWS). Ripples are very evident, even in conditions of using LPF at the level of 40 Hz. Although the first peak is cut off in the frequency spectrum, the second peak at about 100 Hz is present.

Existence of rhythmicity of the cellular discharges is apparent also during visual evaluation of the EEG record.

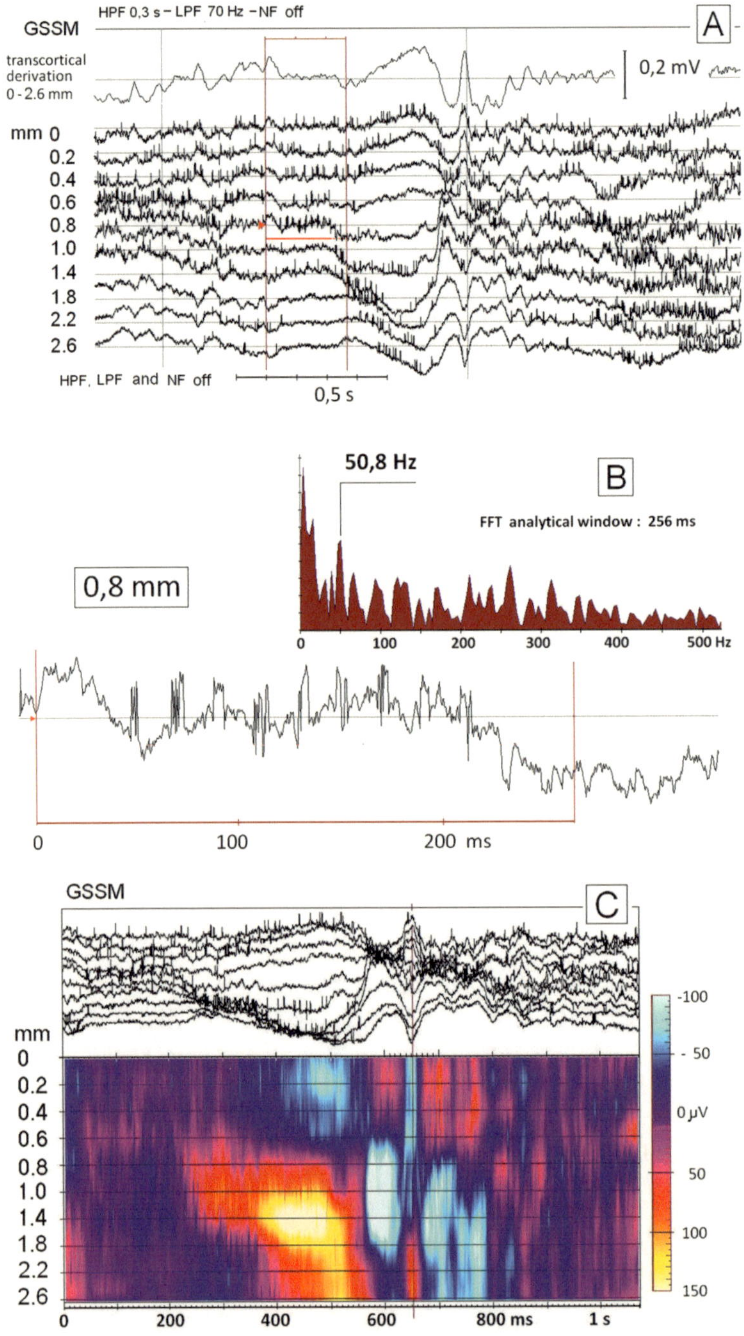

Figure 5.
(A,B,C). Intracortical composition of the bioelectrical patterns coexisting during appearance of the spontaneous discharge of the complex of slow wave and spike, appearing in conditions of IME.

Figure 4(A-C) illustrates results of evaluation of the selected fragment of the IcEEG recorded 3 weeks after electrode implantation. This fragment represents pattern of cortical activity at the stage of slow wave sleep with a tendency of transferring to REM sleep.

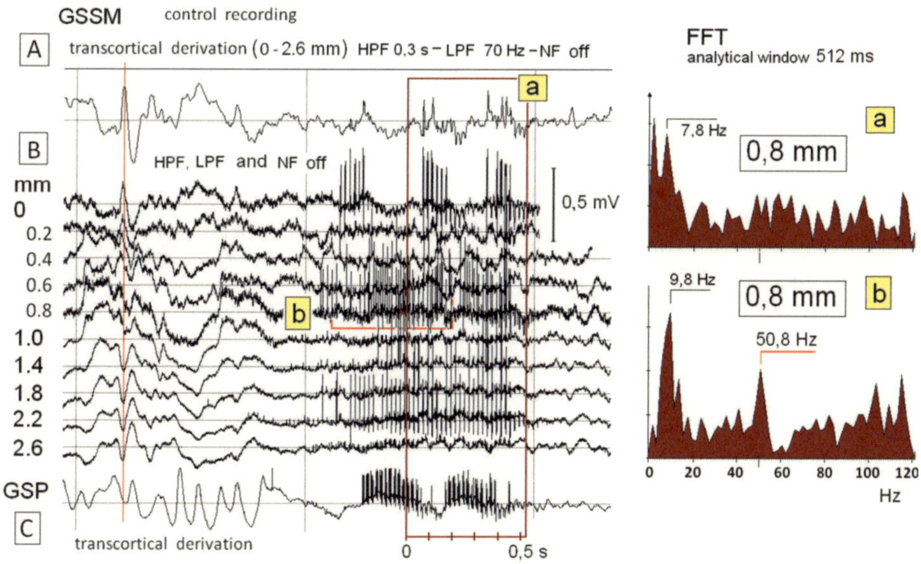

Figure 6.
Illustration of independency of appearance of the EEG spike and cellutar discharges and generalization of discharges in different cortical areas: dischages are present in GSSM as well as GSP records.

Figure 4A illustrates existence of cellular discharges not only in the association cortex (GSSM) but also in somatosensory cortex (GSP). Interestingly, the distribution of these discharges in the somatosensory cortex appears to be independent of the pattern of activity observed in the GSSM. The first channel: transcortical derivation (between the surface and deep electrode: 0–2.6 mm) presents cortical ripples appearing with the intensity much lower in comparison to the deep cortical layers. **Figure 4B** presents the global pattern of the cortical discharges seen after superimposition of all patterns of the cortical activity of EEG fragment indicated on the EEG record. The number of complex structures of the bursts of discharges is about 25 during the period of 512 msec. This is in agreement with the presence of frequency peak seen in the results of FFT evaluation of the EEG record—at the frequency of 46.9 Hz (**Figure 4C**). This peak is absent in conditions of using notch filter (NF on) during EEG recording.

Figure 5(A-C) illustrates appearance of the spontaneous spike following slow wave recorded in conditions of IME. Both, slow wave and spike are with phase reversal between surface and deep structures of neocortex—negative on the surface. Numerous scattered cellutar spikes can be observed across all cortical layers, indicating cortical activity. Although, there are no high amplitude discharges present in the recorded data. However, transient 50 Hz rhythmic activity is present, especially at the level of 0.8 mm (**Figure 5B**), spreading in deeper and more superficial derivations during development of deep intracortical positivity of the slow wave. Exact evaluation of the intracortical localization of the functional elements appearing during development of the surface negative spike is possible during presentation of this IcEEG fragment as a spatio-temporal map (**Figure 5C**). Presence of the surface negative spike appears to be a consequence of previously appearing intracortical negativity, mainly at the depth of 0.8–1.4 mm.

Figure 6 illustrates transient appearance of the 50 Hz rhythm in frequency spectrum of the burst of high amplitude discharges appearing, during control recording after testing brain activity in conditions of PME. During the burst, there is a tendency

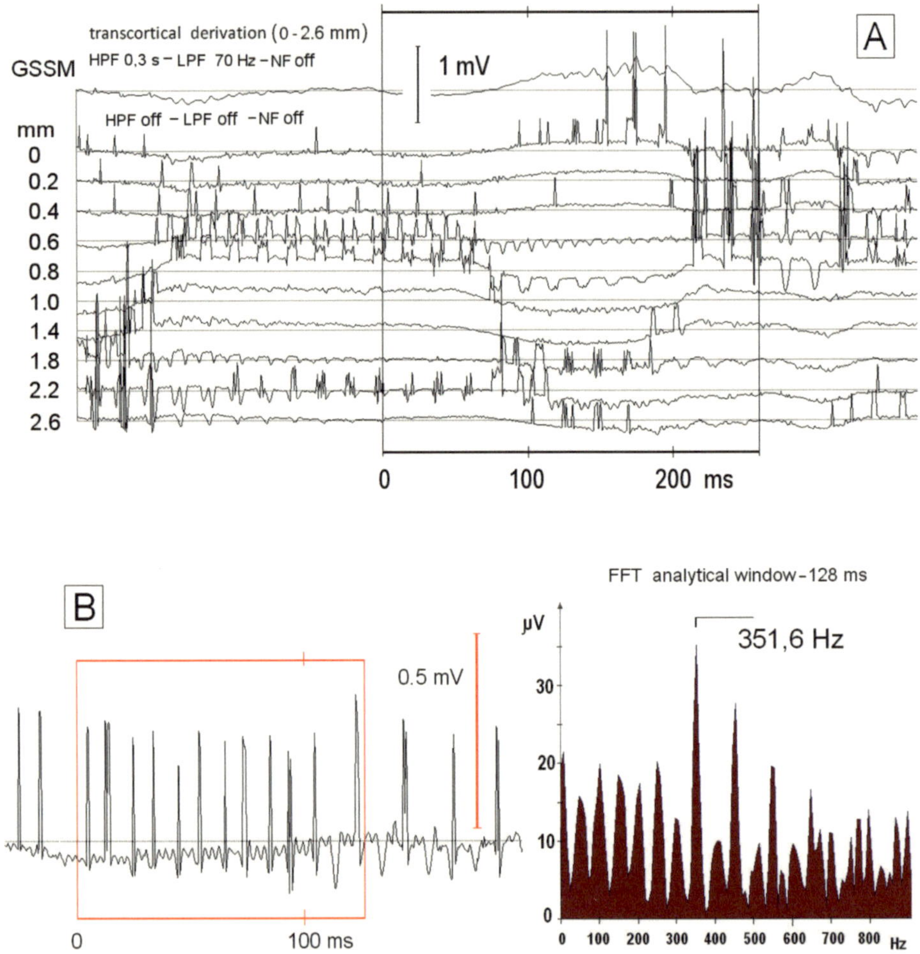

Figure 7.
(A,B). Patterns of the components of selected IcEEG samples, participating in formation of groups of the cortical cellular discharges. (B) illustrates possibility of identification of the origin of high frequency oscillations - frequency about 350 Hz - during visual evaluation of EEG records.

for the pattern of IcEEG to become desynchronized. The burst is preceded by single EEG spike.

Figure 7(**A, B**) illustrates composition of the bioelectrical patterns that reflect the functional states of the elements within the intracortical cellular network engaged in producing HFOs. These patterns exhibit various frequencies, with a basic rhythm of approximately 50/s of the complexes of one or two groups of spikes of low and high amplitudes, lasting about 10 ms. The highest frequencies observed in the low amplitude rhythmic activity are about 300/s.

Figure 7B illustrates a selected sample of EEG with rhythmic high amplitude spikes. The spikes, or groups of spikes, are spaced approximately 10 ms apart, creating a regular pattern. Additionally, there is a presence of fast, low amplitude waves (about three waves in a period of 10 msec.). The analytical system identifies two rhythmic patterns in the EEG data. The first pattern has leading frequencies at about 50, 100, 150, 200, 250 Hz, and so on. The second pattern shows the first peak at

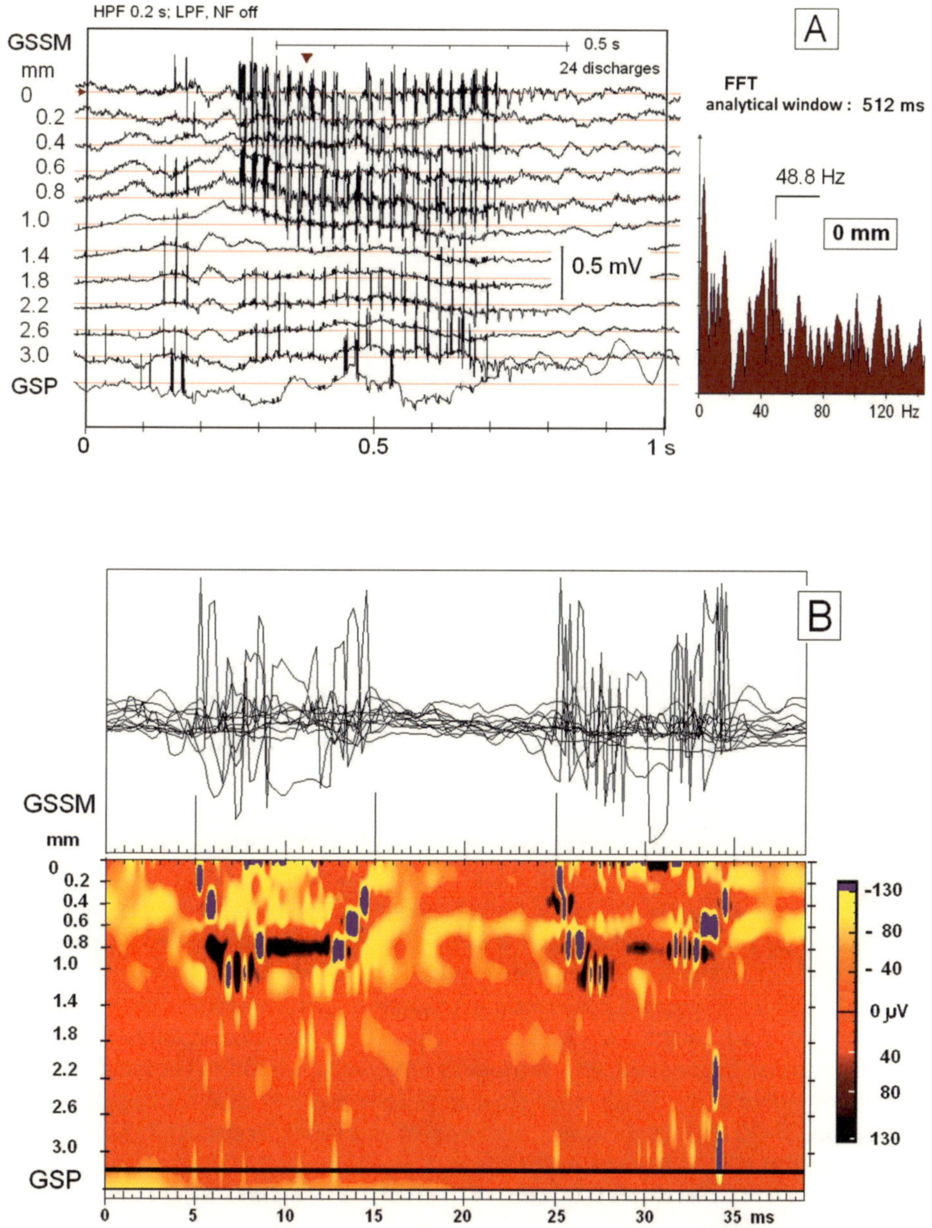

Figure 8.
(A,B). Results of analysis of the spatio-temporal organization of the composition of the elements creating group of cellutar discharges. Selected fragment is indicated on the IcEEG record illustrated in **Figure 8(A)**.

351.6 Hz. These frequency components represent the recurring rhythms observed in the recorded EEG signal. The compositions of these elements are more precisely presented in **Figure 8(A, B)**.

Figure 8(A, B) illustrates presence of the group of complexes of spikes (about 24 groups in a period of 500 msec.), appearing especially in superficial cortical layers. The leading frequency of the components in the frequency spectrum is 48.8 Hz

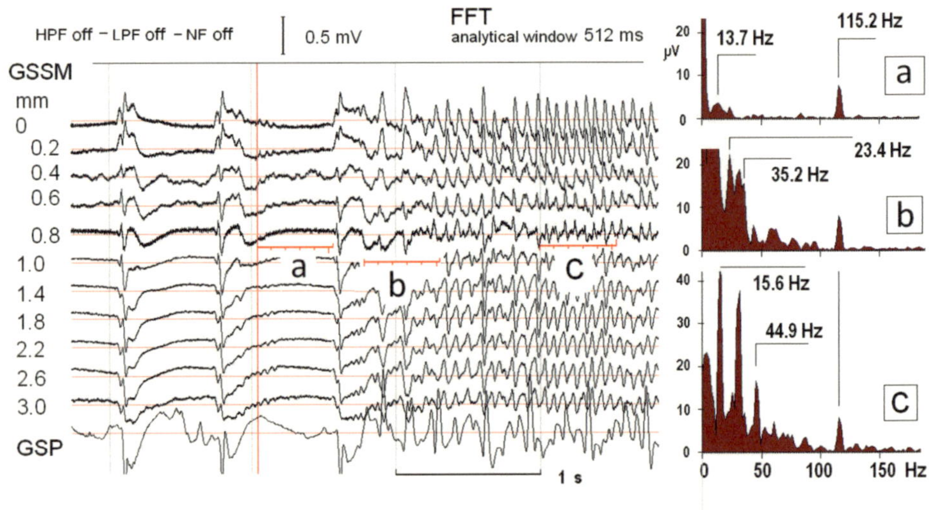

Figure 9.
Transition of the IcEEG pattern to bioelectrical seizure after epicortical injection of penicillin in conditions of general anaesthesia (PME).

(in derivation 0 mm), cohesive with the number of the group of spikes detected during visual evaluation of the EEG record.

Figure 8B presents spatio-temporal composition of the elements within the circuits of the two groups of spikes and existence of low amplitude fast oscillation (between groups of spikes).

Figure 9 illustrates onset of a bioelectrical seizure in the cortical structure of the same animal. The seizure is recorded after the epicortical administration of penicillin, while the animal is under general anesthesia caused by pentobarbital. There are no signs of high amplitude discharges. It may be suspected, that the electrical noise dominating in channels 0 to 0.8 mm reflects 50 Hz artifacts caused by the widespread electrical field or muscular (EMG-electromyographic) artifact. However, the results obtained from the frequency analysis (FFT) clearly illustrate the organization of the observed pattern. In fragment (b), frequency ranges correspond to the frequencies of waves observed in the EEG record (low amplitude waves seen at the beginning of the seizure (20–30 Hz). Surprisingly, fast oscillations (peak frequency 115.2 Hz) are detected at all stages (a, b, c) of analysis.

Figure 10(A-C) illustrates fragment of the EEG record confirming existence of the complex, basically 50 Hz pattern of cellular activity recorded in another animal, after epicortical injection of penicillin. The effects of this procedure were tested in conditions of deep anesthesia, after administration of pentobarbital.

Figure 10A illustrates fragment of the IcEEG record, typical for EEG patterns existing between bioelectrical seizures: existence of single, high amplitude surface negative sharp waves, with suppression of EEG rhythmic activity between their discharges. Comparison of intracortical, vertical distribution of the patterns of discharges illustrates existence of phase reversal of the main, surface negative component (negativity dominates in two superficial derivations – from the depth 0 and 0.2 mm, with clear positivity, especially at the levels of 1.4, 1.8, and 2.2 mm). This findings confirm the probability that localization of this electrode reflects activity of the cortical cells with localizations at the supra-granular (L3), granular L4, and

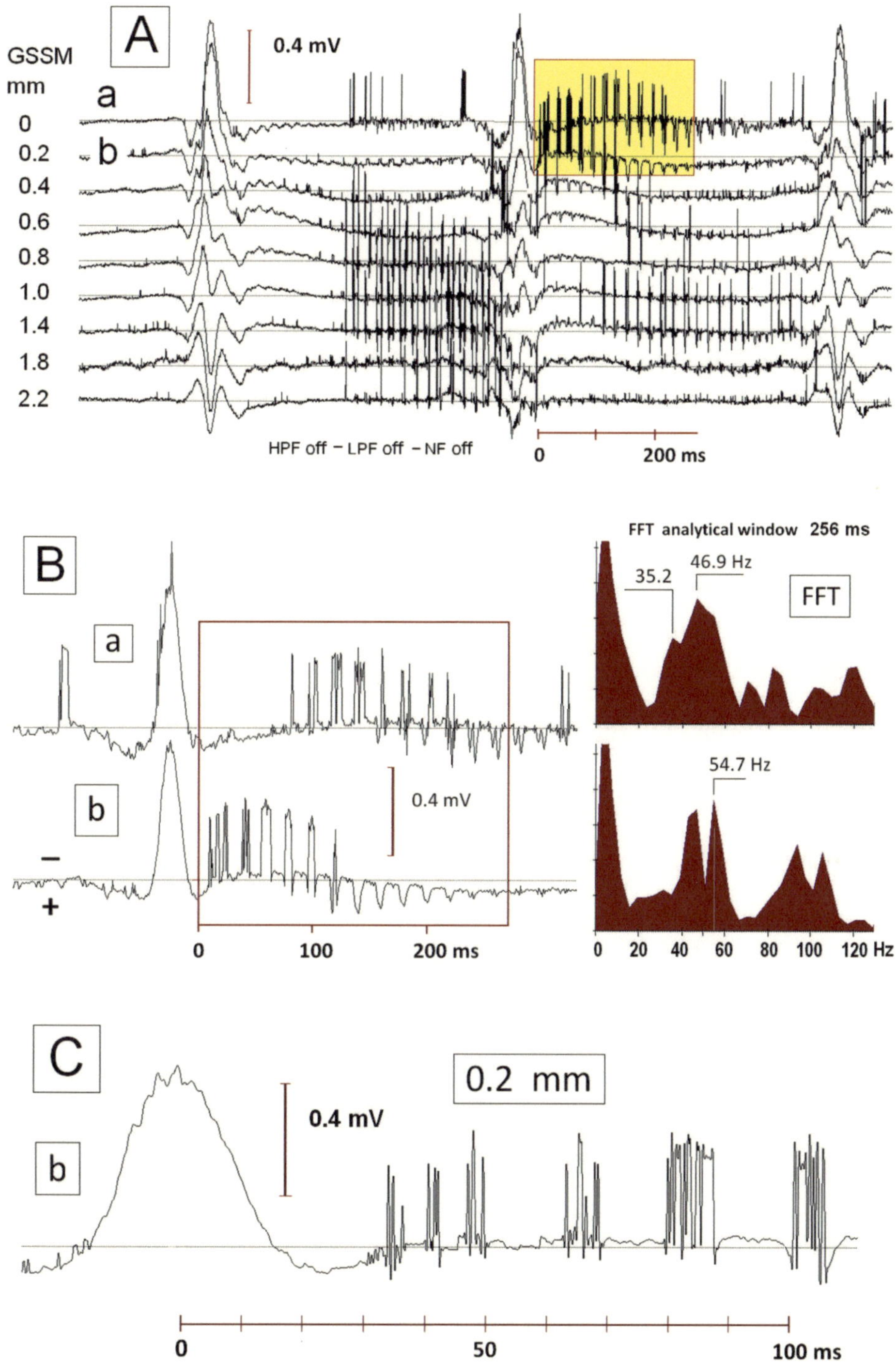

Figure 10.
(A,B,C). Cellular and EEG patterns recorded between consecutive epileptiform seizures in anaesthetized animal (PME).

infra-granular (L5 and L6) layers of the cerebral cortex. Groups of cellular discharges are present between discharges of sharp waves.

Figure 10B illustrates more accurately compositions of the EEG fragment indicated on the record presented in **Figure 10A**: derivations 0 mm (a) and 0.2 mm (b). The main frequencies reflecting cellular activity are between 40 and 60 Hz. **Figure 10C** [b] illustrates existence of groups of numerous spikes reflected as single waves in records presented in **Figure 10B** [b].

4. Conclusion

The presented results of this investigation illustrate complexity of the process of epileptogenic functional reorganization of the cortical activity. Presented illustrations suggest possibility of existence of the EEG pattern reflecting functional state of the intracortical cellular network, relatively independent from the cellular activity of the neuronal systems engaged in formation of the conventional, normal, and abnormal EEG patterns. Functional patterns reflecting activation of this system are presented in wide frequency spectrum of the cortical electrical activity: within the range of gamma and higher frequencies (HFOs), with the basic frequency of activity in gamma frequency range (40–60 Hz). Interdisciplinary approach is necessary in explaining the background and significance of demonstrated phenomenon.

Acknowledgements

The author thanks his wife, Barbara Kosicka-Sobieszek PhD for cooperation in preparation of this manuscript.

Author note

This research was supported by the Committee for Scientific Research, Republic of Poland, grant 4-T11E-008-22.

Author details

Aleksander Sobieszek
Independent Scientist, Warszawa, Poland

*Address all correspondence to: so.aleks.warsaw@gmail.com

References

[1] Gotman J. Oh surprise! Fast ripples on scalp EEG. Clinical Neurophysiology. 2018;**129**:1449-1450

[2] Zijlmans M, Worell GA, Dümpelmann M, Stieglitz T, Barborica A, Heers M, et al. How to record high-frequency oscillations in epilepsy: A practical guideline. Epilepsia. 2017;**58**(8):1305-1315

[3] von Ellenrieder N, Dubeau F, Gotman J, Frauscher B. Physiological and pathological high-frequency oscillations have distinct sleep-homeostatic properties. Neuroimage: Clinical. 2017;**14**:566-573

[4] Marcus EM. Experimental models of petit mal epilepsy. In: Purpura DP, Penry KJ, Woodbury DM, Tower DB, Walted RD, editors. Experimental Models of Epilepsy – A Manual for the Laboratory Worker. New York: Raven Press; 1972. pp. 113-146

[5] Sobieszek A. P16-T early signs of transformation of neocortical activity to epileptiform patterns in experimental model of epilepsy. Clinical Neurophysiology. 2019;**130**(Issue 7):e42-e43. DOI: 10.1016/j.clinph.2019.04.379

Chapter 2

Study on Gut Microbiota in Children with Cerebral Palsy and Epilepsy

Congfu Huang and Defeng Cai

Abstract

Compared to children with cerebral palsy (CP), children with both CP and concurrent epilepsy (CPE) have more severe gastrointestinal symptoms, such as functional constipation (FC), and are more prone to recurrent infections. Our previous study found that these children have gut microbiota (GM) disorders, which are significantly related to the gastrointestinal symptoms and immune functions. The children with CPE also has altered oral microbiota (OM), which is consistent with the change of GM. In addition, the change of OM and GM has potential impact on the occurrence of clinical diseases such as periodontitis, dental caries and malnutrition. In our previous study, it was also found that the abundance of butyric acid- and lactic acid-producing bacteria in the GM of children who have CPE with liquid food in their diet decreased significantly, while the abundance of opportunistic pathogenic bacteria increased significantly. After the butyric acid-, lactic acid-producing probiotics and dietary fibers were administered by us to treat the FC in children with CPE, the FC improved significantly, and the abundance of butyric acid- and lactic acid-producing bacteria in the intestine increased.

Keywords: cerebral palsy with epilepsy, gut microbiota, oral microbiota, probiotics, dietary fiber

1. Introduction

Cerebral palsy (CP) is a group of neurological disorders that are caused by damage to the developing brain in fetuses or infants, which leads to permanent impairment of cerebral motor functions and impairment of abilities to maintain balance and posture [1]. Besides impaired cognitive function development, patients with CP often have many other co-occurring cerebral neurological disorders, such as epilepsy which has an incidence of 35–62% with an average of 43% in patients with CP [2]. The onset of concurrent epilepsy (CPE) disease is usually in infancy or early childhood, with more than half of CPE first appearing before 1 year old and more than 92% of CPE first occurring before 4 years old [2–6]. The incidence of epilepsy in patients with CP is five times that of normal children without CP [7]. The main risk factors for epilepsy in children with CP include neonatal convulsions, low birth weight, intracranial hemorrhage, gray and white matter lesions caused by brain damage, and brain structure malformations [8, 9]. The incidence of CPE is also related to the types of CP, with most of the CPE occurring in patients with spastic CP which has a younger age of onset as well [10–12]. The occurrence of epileptic seizures might increase brain damage in CPE patients, impairing cognitive and motor function development, affecting directly the treatment outcomes and prognosis in patients with CPE, and significantly decreasing the life quality of the patient's family members [3, 6, 13]. Patients with CPE have a higher incidence of paralysis in the three or four limbs, with a more severe CP (grade IV and grade V palsies) as well [14]. The cognitive, movement, and behavioral difficulties are increased in CPE patients due to the existence of epilepsy [15, 16]. The epileptic seizures can be controlled well by anti-epileptic medications in some of the children with CPE. Some patients might even develop resistance to the anti-epileptic drugs, leading to the development of intractable epilepsy [17, 18]. The incidence of obstructive sleep apnoea (OSA) is also higher in children with CPE compared to children with only CP [18]. As a result, early and sustainable control of the occurrence of epileptic seizures in CPE patients directly affects the long-term prognosis of these patients.

There are often common pathogenesis and etiology shared between epilepsy and CP. The risk factors for epilepsy and CP can be divided into three types: 1. Prenatal factors: such as consanguineous marriages, multiple pregnancies, intrauterine infections, intrauterine growth retardation, and history of use of medications in pregnant women, etc. [19]. 2. Perinatal factors: such as placenta previa, perinatal asphyxia, premature infant, placental abruption, and infant of low birth weight, etc. [20]. 3. Postnatal factors: such as neonatal hyperbilirubinemia and non-infectious or infectious diseases, etc. In recent years, with the advances in medicines and technologies, many premature infants or infants with very low birth weights can survive. But the problems of the occurrence of movement disorders, cognitive disorders, sensory disorders, cognitive abnormalities, and learning disabilities in these premature babies have gradually come into the picture [21].

About 80–90% of patients with CP have some gastrointestinal disorders, such as constipation, dysphagia, hypersalivation, and gastroesophageal reflux, among which the incidence of functional constipation (FC) reaches 26–74% [22, 23]. The incidence of FC is even higher in patients with CPE, which might reach 100% in some studies, with a more frequent occurrence of abdominal distensions and upper gastrointestinal tract hemorrhage, etc. in CPE patients [24–26]. These gastrointestinal disorders significantly affect CPE patients physically, socially, and emotionally, decreasing the quality of life in children with CPE [27, 28]. The alteration of gut microbiota (GM), on the other hand, can affect gastrointestinal functions. Our studies have found that there is a unique composition of gastrointestinal microbiota in patients with CPE [24–26, 29].

2. The characteristics of the composition of digestive tract microbiota in CPE patients

2.1 The characteristics of GM in CPE patients

The principal component analysis (PCA) study showed that there is a separation of microorganisms in GM in the specimens from CPE patients and healthy individuals. The isolated microorganisms include *Bacteroides*, *Bifidobacterium*, *Prevotella*,

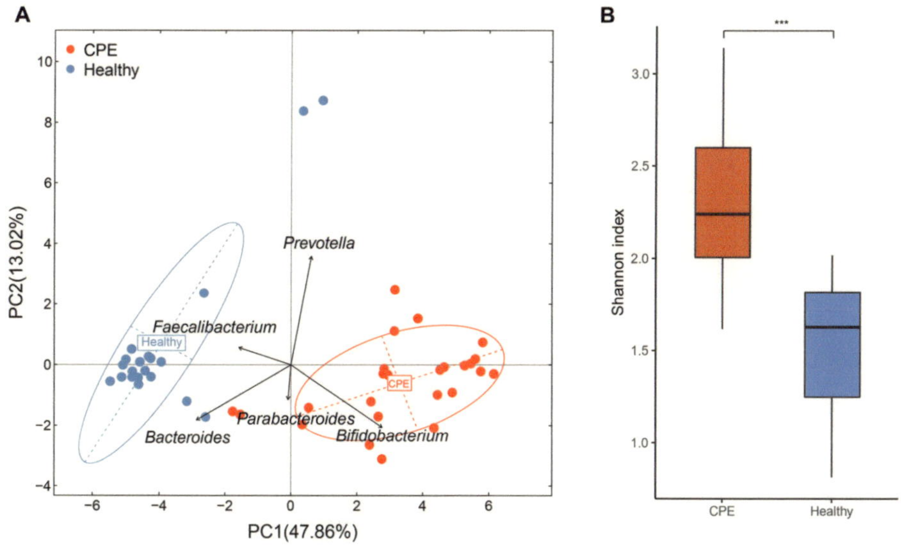

Figure 1.
(A) PCA of CPE patients and healthy individuals. (B) Alpha diversity of CPE patients and healthy individuals.

Faecalibacterium, and *Parabacteroides* (**Figure 1A**). Besides, the diversity of microorganisms and the Shannon index in the CPE patients group are higher compared to that in the healthy individual's group (**Figure 1B**).

Compared to healthy children, there is a significant alteration in GM in CPE patients [24, 25]. The relative abundance of *Actinomycetes* significantly increases while the relative abundance of *Bacteroides* significantly decreases in the CPE patients at the phyla level. On the other hand, at the Genus level, the relative abundance of the beneficial bacteria *Bifidobacterium* significantly increases, and the relative abundance of the opportunistic bacteria such as *Parabacteroides*, *Enterococcus*, and *Streptococcus* increases as well, but the relative abundance of butyric acid-producing bacteria such as *Bacteroides*, *Faecalibacterium*, *Ruminococcus*, and *Roseburia* significantly decreases. The above changes in GM can lead to chronic inflammations in the intestines which is closely related to gastrointestinal functional disorders such as FC. After the KEGG annotation and function enrichment analysis, it can be seen that the xenobiotics metabolism, immune system diseases, and neurodegenerative diseases are increased in CPE patients. In contrast, the functional categories related to the biosynthesis of secondary metabolites are reduced. Furthermore, the increased risk of neurodegenerative diseases is mainly attributed to *Streptococcus*, while the increased risk of immune system diseases is associated with enriched *Akkermansia* in CPE patients (**Figure 2**).

2.2 The association study on GM and OM in CPE patients

There are usually many oral diseases appearing in the patients with CP, such as periodontitis, and dental caries [30, 31]. The previous studies have also shown that the abundance of *Fusobacterium nucleatum* and *Porphyromonas gingivalis* were significantly elevated in the oral cavity of CP patients [32, 33], which induces the alteration of GM through different approaches and leads to gastrointestinal functional disorders such as FC [34–36]. It was found through our surveys that 26 out of 27 (96.30%) CPE patients suffered from periodontitis, while 22 patients (81.48%) suffered from

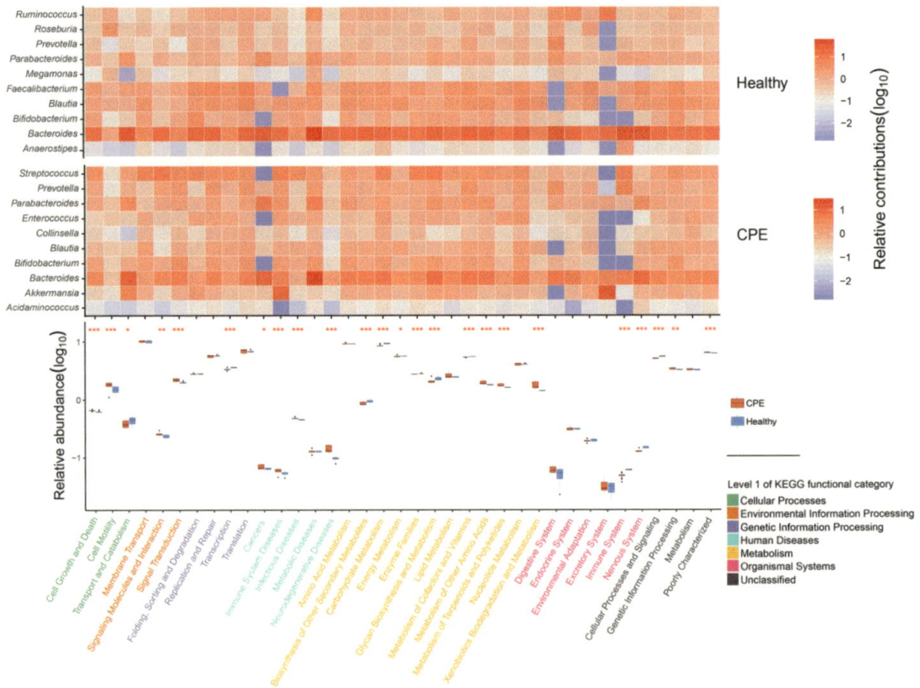

Figure 2.
Composition and functional categories of GM.

various degrees of dental caries and 11 patients (40.74%) developed intractable constipation [28]. The bacterial plaques on the gingiva in CPE patients might enter the stomach and intestines through the enteral pathway (e.g. through ingestion and swallowing) and the bloodstream route (e.g. invading the capillaries in the endodontic through the root canal). Thus, acid-tolerant bacteria might enter and colonize the stomach and intestines, which can lead to the alteration of GM and chronic intestinal inflammations. It might also induce developmental defects in the brain, neuroinflammation, and neurodegenerative diseases through the vagus nerve route (leading to neurotransmitters disorders, e.g. GABA and acetylcholine), tryptophan metabolism (e.g. quinolinic acid and kynurenic acid) and microbial metabolism disorders (e.g. SCFA and peptidoglycan), which aggravates the neurological symptoms in the CP patients [37].

We also discovered that the first three dominant bacteria in oral microbiota (OM) in CPE patients are *Prevotella*, *Fusobacterium*, and *Neisseria*, which are potentially linked to dental caries, periodontitis, and malnutritions in CPE patients [29]. In addition, there is a positive correlation between the disorders' frequency and the levels of *Solobacterium*, *Lachnoanaerobaculum*, *Corynebacterium*, and *Veillonella* in the OM in the CPE patients. On the contrary, the levels of *Actinomyces*, *Corynebacterium*, *Leptotrichia*, and *Veillonella* correlated negatively with the spasm frequency. As for GM, the frequency of disorders is associated positively with *Alloprevotella* and *Blautia*, but negatively with *Alistipes* and *Clostridium_XVIII*. In addition, the spasm frequency is in positive association with *Senegalimassilia*, *Staphylococcus*, *Actinomyces*, and *Bacillus*, but in a negative association with *Sutterella* and *Victivallis*. Overall,

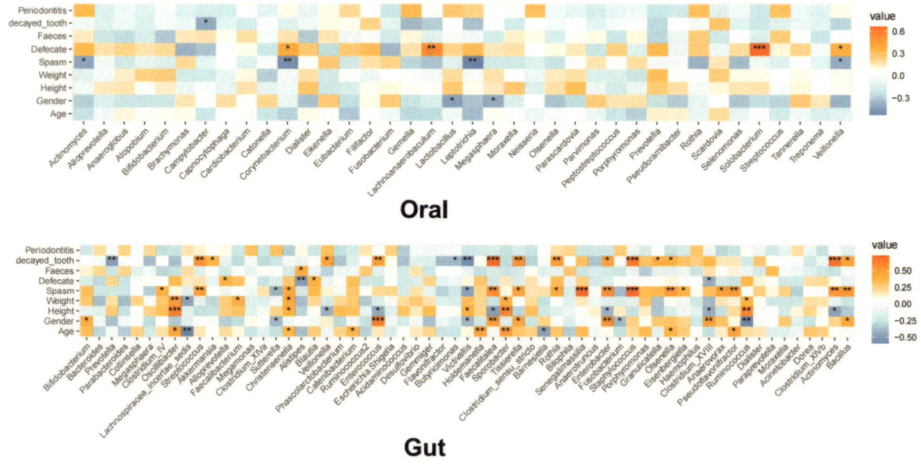

Figure 3.
Association between OM/GM and clinical manifestations.

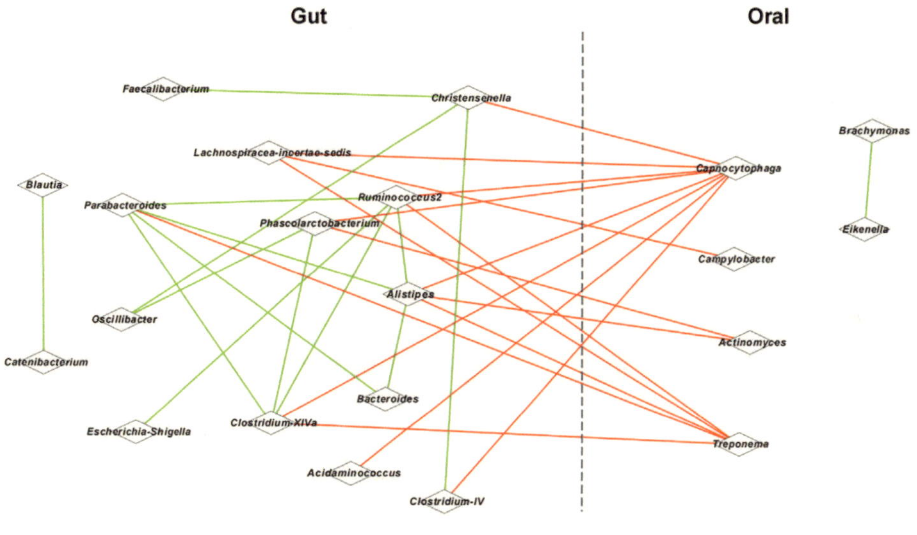

Figure 4.
Association between OM and GM.

these findings suggest that there is a significant association between the frequency of disorders and spasms and OM and GM. However, the mechanisms behind this should still be further explored (**Figure 3**).

Given the significant correlation between disorder/spasm frequency and oral/GM, we further conducted another association analysis for OM and GM. Based on the statistical analysis using Spearman's coefficient ($P < 0.05$), it was shown that there is a positive correlation between oral *Capnocytophaga* and intestinal *Christensenella*, Clostridium-IV. A positive correlation is also identified between oral *Campylobacter* and intestinal *Lachnospiracea-incertaesedis*, between oral *Actinomyces* and intestinal *Phascolarctobacterium* and *Alistipes*, as well as between oral *Treponema* and intestinal *Clostridium-XlVa*, *Parabacteroides* and *Alistipes* (**Figure 4**).

2.3 The diet and GM in CPE patients

Diet is an important factor that affects the composition and function of GM. As we know, GM plays a key role in maintaining the normal functions of the gastrointestinal tract, and the alteration of GM is involved in the development and pathogenesis of functional gastrointestinal disorders. It was also found that most of the CPE patients who ingested liquid food in their diet suffered from FC. The intestinal tract of these patients was enriched with opportunistic pathogenic bacteria such as *Collinsella*, *Alistipes*, and *Eggerthella*. In addition, the abundance of *Bifidobacterium* was significantly increased in the patients fed with dairy products. Meanwhile, the intestinal tract in patients fed with a regular diet was enriched with the butyric acid-producing bacteria which are also found in the healthy population, such as the *Lachnoclostridium*, *Dorea*, *Ruminococcus*, *Faecalibacterium*, *Roseburia*, and *Coprococcus*, while the abundance of *Prevotella* for carbohydrate degradation was significantly increased in this group of patients as well [26] (**Table 1**). The above results suggest that the barrier of intestinal mucosa was damaged in the CPE patients who had a liquid diet, resulting in a significantly higher incidence of gastrointestinal disorders such as FC.

2.4 Intervention of FC in CPE patients with probiotics and dietary fibers

Dietary fibers are carbohydrates that can not be digested by humans, which are also the fermentation substrate for the intestinal normal microbiota [38]. Therefore, the dietary fibers can promote the proliferation of probiotics, especially

Regular diet group			**Liquid diet group**		
The first 15 dominant bacteria	**Mean value (%)**	**SD (%)**	**The first 15 dominant bacteria**	**Mean value (%)**	**SD (%)**
Prevotella	25.85	26.11	*Bifidobacterium*	24.93	15.60
Bifidobacterium	12.95	17.04	*Bacteroides*	12.13	11.31
Bacteroides	8.45	8.91	*Enterococcus*	6.15	16.59
Parabacteroides	3.92	7.47	*Parabacteroides*	5.13	4.92
Streptococcus	2.79	3.24	*Collinsella*	4.51	3.96
Faecalibacterium	2.32	2.19	*Prevotella*	3.61	7.38
Collinsella	2.15	4.05	*Streptococcus*	2.71	3.65
Sutterella	1.68	1.94	*Akkermansia*	2.02	2.51
Acidaminococcus	1.35	3.95	*Megasphaera*	1.79	3.10
Roseburia	1.35	1.78	*Blautia*	1.48	2.79
Megasphaera	1.33	3.87	*Alistipes*	1.45	2.29
Alloprevotella	1.32	1.82	*Eubacterium*	1.40	4.45
Enterococcus	1.13	2.78	*Faecalibacterium*	1.16	2.24
Catenibacterium	1.02	1.71	*Desulfovibrio*	0.87	1.97
Megamonas	1.02	3.13	*Sutterella*	1.68	1.94

Table 1.
The first 15 dominant bacteria in the regular diet group and the liquid diet group.

the *Lactobacillus* and *Bifidobacterium* [39], and inhibit the growth of opportunistic pathogenic bacteria or harmful bacteria [40]. Probiotics have a similar effect with dietary fibers. For example, the lactic acid-producing probiotics bacteria can produce some metabolites (e.g. short chain fatty acids, SCFAs) which can promote the intestinal peristalsis and the secretions from the intestinal mucosa, lowering the intestinal pH, acidifying the intestinal tract environment, thus improving constipation. Also, the propionic acid and the butyric acid in the SCFAs can induce the secretions of sIgA from the plasma cells in the lamina propria in the intestinal mucosa, and also induce the development and differentiation of Treg cells, and decrease the occurrence of mucosal inflammations, and promote the expression of tight-junction proteins, and maintain the barrier of intestinal mucosa [41].

Compound dietary fiber powders (contain psyllium cylindrical shell powder, resistant dextrin, apple pectin, Konjac powder, and 20 g of dietary fiber complex is contained in each pack), lactic acid-producing complex probiotics (contain *Lactobacillus rhamnosus*, *Lactobacillus acidophilus*, *Lactobacillus paracei*, *Lactobacillus plantarum*, *Bifidobacterium lactis*, sorbitol, fructooligosaccharide, xylooligosaccharides, and viable bacteria ≥18 billion CFUs per pack) and butyric acid-producing probiotics (each pack contains viable *Clostridium butyricum* bacteria ≥1.0 × 107 CFUs/g, viable *Bifidobacterium* bacteria ≥1.0 × 106 CFUs/g) were administered for the intervention of FC in the CPE patients, with 1-month administration of compound dietary fiber powders and 6 months administration of lactic acid-producing complex probiotics and butyric acid-producing probiotics [42]. FC was relieved in all of the CPE patients after the intervention course, with improved abdominal distensions and nutritional conditions and increased body weight in some of the CPE patients (**Figure 5**).

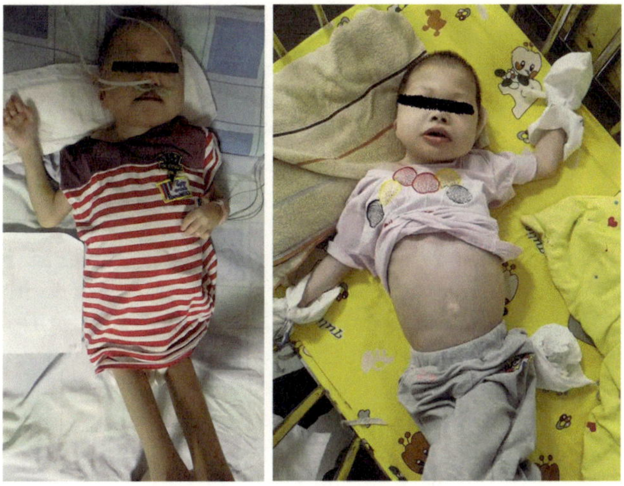

Figure 5.
Comparison before and after treatment in a child with CPE (2019.10.09 vs. 2020.03.26. Their body weights were 9.8 and 11.5 kg, respectively). Week 1: Open plug dew seven capsules/week (exhaust), defecation seven times/week (forming hard stool), serious abdominal distension; Week 2: Open plug dew zero capsules/week, defecation seven times/week (forming hard stool), abdominal distension significantly reduced; Week 3: Open plug dew zero capsules/week, defecation seven times/week (forming hard stool), slight abdominal distension; Week 4: Open plug dew zero capsules/week, defecation seven times/week (forming soft stool), abdominal distension disappeared; Week 24: Open plug dew zero capsules/week, defecation seven times/week (forming soft stool), abdominal distension disappeared. Note: The above pictures of children have been authorized and approved by the guardian of Longgang district Social Welfare Center.

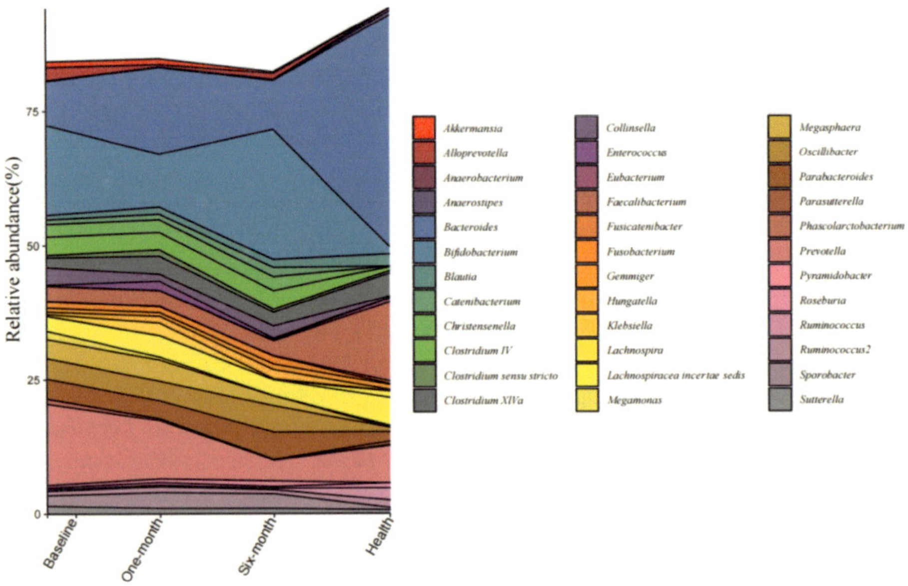

Figure 6.
Changes in the levels and abundance of bacterial genus before and after the intervention.

The abundance of dominant GM in the Genus level has changed before and after the intervention. The abundance of some bacterial genus continued to drop after the intervention, such as the *Prevotella*, *Collinsella*, *Sutterella* and *Megamonas*. The abundance of some bacterial genus was increased after the intervention for 1 month, but was decreased after the intervention for 6 months, such as the *Bacteroides*, *Faecalibacterium* and *Lachnospiracea-incertaesedis*. The abundance of some bacterial genus was decreased after the intervention for 1 month, but was raised after the intervention for 6 months, such as the *Bifidobacterium*, *Oscillibacter* and *Parabacteroides* (**Figure 6**). The above results suggest that both the compound dietary fiber powders and the probiotics products should be administered for 6 months, which should exert a more sustaining effect in restoring the composition of GM.

Considering the diet being the most significant factor affecting the composition of GM, which also causes the largest interference on the outcomes of therapeutic interventions. In this study, the composition of GM in the CPE patients with different diets in different diet groups varied significantly. Therefore, a stratified statistical analysis was also conducted. The results showed that the abundance of intestinal *Lactobacillus* and *Clostridium* displayed an increasing trend in the CPE patients with regular diet after the intervention, but the increase is not statistically significant. The abundance of *Bifidobacterium* was decreased after the 1-month intervention and was increased again after the 6-month intervention in the CPE patients with regular diet (**Table 2**). The abundance of the above three bacteria all changed statistically significantly in the CPE patients with liquid diet after the intervention: the abundance of intestinal *Lactobacillus* and *Clostridium* showed a statistically significant increase after the intervention. The abundance of *Bifidobacterium* was decreased after the 1-month intervention and was increased statistically significantly after the 6-month intervention in the CPE patients with liquid diet (**Table 3**). The above results suggest that the supplementation of probiotics products can help in raising the abundance of relevant intestinal microflora bacteria in the CPE patients, while the CPE patients in the liquid

	Before intervention	After intervention for 1 month	After intervention for 6 months	P value (0 vs. 1)	P value (0 vs. 6)
Lactobacillus	**0.0661 ± 0.0997**	**0.1339 ± 0.1055**	**0.1407 ± 0.1502**	**0.596**	**0.158**
Bifidobacterium	**8.8179 ± 16.6314**	**5.6035 ± 5.7671**	**7.3992 ± 4.3123**	**0.077**	**0.111**
Clostridium	**7.9263 ± 4.6011**	**8.7353 ± 2.7794**	**8.2450 ± 3.1322**	**0.791**	**1**
Clostridium_IV	5.7130 ± 3.9603	4.1067 ± 1.6176	4.4595 ± 1.7363	0.377	0.596
Clostridium_XIVa	1.5597 ± 1.0576	3.5114 ± 1.1483	2.6450 ± 1.4694	0.005	0.185
Clostridium_sensu_stricto	0.3380 ± 0.4398	0.5299 ± 0.2232	0.6509 ± 0.5816	0.077	0.093
Clostridium_XIVb	0.1593 ± 0.1655	0.1817 ± 0.1269	0.1598 ± 0.0903	0.377	0.536
Clostridium_XVIII	0.1558 ± 0.1678	0.4053 ± 0.2265	0.3298 ± 0.6121	0.017	0.659

Table 2.
Changes in the abundance of probiotics bacteria in feces before and after the intervention in the CPE patients in the regular diet group (mean ± SD, %).

	Before intervention	After intervention for 1 month	After intervention for 6 months	P value (0 vs. 1)	P value (0 vs. 6)
Lactobacillus	**0.0332 ± 0.0522**	**0.1304 ± 0.1381**	**0.5156 ± 0.7946**	**0.001**	**0.000**
Bifidobacterium	**20.6816 ± 16.635**	**12.0629 ± 7.2618**	**32.3191 ± 18.706**	**0.307**	**0.047**
Clostridium	**4.4997 ± 3.3378**	**6.6342 ± 2.5942**	**5.1066 ± 1.4805**	**0.033**	**0.308**
Clostridium_IV	2.2163 ± 2.3703	2.6537 ± 1.2842	2.9365 ± 1.1905	0.137	0.085
Clostridium_sensu_stricto	0.5072 ± 0.8519	1.5424 ± 1.6814	0.4944 ± 0.4986	0.001	0.152
Clostridium_XIVa	1.5749 ± 1.1317	2.1135 ± 0.9210	1.6305 ± 0.5925	0.080	0.381
Clostridium_XIVb	0.1267 ± 0.1927	0.1195 ± 0.0870	0.1324 ± 0.0822	0.199	0.085
Clostridium_XVIII	0.0722 ± 0.1143	0.2047 ± 0.1683	0.0747 ± 0.0525	0.000	0.090

Table 3.
Changes in the abundance of probiotics bacteria in feces before and after the intervention in the CPE patients in the liquid diet group (mean ± SD, %).

diet group showed a sustaining response to the therapeutic intervention and showed a better response compared to the CPE patients in the regular diet group.

3. Conclusion

CPE patients often have concurrent functional gastrointestinal disorders, especially FC, which have a unique composition of digestive tract microbiota as well. The altered OM can then enter the gastrointestinal tract through different routes, leading to disordered GM which produces metabolites that can cause damage to the barrier function of the intestinal mucosa, resulting in chronic intestinal inflammations that are able to induce or aggravate FC. This can also affect brain functions through the gut-brain axis (GBA). Based on the therapeutic target of GM in CPE patients, the administration of specific probiotics bacteria and dietary fiber products was able to improve FC, restoring some of the composition and function of GM (e.g. the abundance of the butyric acid-producing and lactic acid-producing bacteria showed an increase). This approach to interventions could also improve the quality of sleep and improve the absorption of nutrients and metabolic conditions in CPE patients. However, whether the mental and neurological symptoms can be improved through the effects of GBA in CPE patients still needs to be further studied in the future.

Acknowledgements

We are thankful for the large amount of work done by the staff at the Longgang District Social Welfare Centre of Shenzhen City and the Longgang District Maternity and Child Healthcare Hospital of Shenzhen City. We also appreciate the funds and support from the Science and Technology Innovation Bureau of Longgang District of Shenzhen City. We also want to thank the BGI Nutrition Precision Co., Ltd. (Shenzhen) for the provision of therapeutic intervention products.

Conflict of interest

All the pictures and tables are original works from the author. We declared that there are no conflicts of interest.

Author details

Congfu Huang[1*] and Defeng Cai[2]

1 Department of Pediatrics, Longgang District Maternity and Child Healthcare Hospital, Shenzhen, China

2 Clinical Laboratory (Pathology) Center, South China Hospital of Shenzhen University, Shenzhen, China

*Address all correspondence to: 78333755@qq.com

References

[1] Chinese Association of Rehabilitation Medicine, China Association of Rehabilitation of Disabled Persons of Children with Cerebral Palsy Specialized Committee, Editorial Committee of Guidelines for Rehabilitation of Rerebral Palsy in China. Guidelines for rehabilitation of cerebral palsy in China (2015): Section 1. Chinese Journal of Rehabilitation Medicine. 2015;**30**(7):747-754. DOI: 10.3969/j.issn.1001-1242.2015.07.028

[2] Zhao Y, Ren YP, Xiao N. Research progress of cerebral palsy combined with epilepsy. Chinese Journal of Physical Medicine and Rehabilitation. 2011;**33**(5):392-394. DOI: 10.3760/cma.j.issn.0254-1424.2011.05.025

[3] Mert GG, Incecik F, Altunbasak S, et al. Factors affecting epilepsy development and epilepsy prognosis in cerebral palsy. Pediatric Neurology. 2011;**45**(2):89-94. DOI:10.1016/j.pediatrneurol.2011.03.001

[4] Novak I, Hines M, Goldsmith S, et al. Clinical prognostic messages from a systematic review on cerebral palsy. Pediatrics. 2012;**130**(5):e1285-e1312. DOI:10.1542/peds.2012-0924

[5] Sellier E, Uldall P, Calado E, et al. Epilepsy and cerebral palsy: characteristics and trends in children born in 1976-1998. European Journal of Paediatric Neurology. 2012;**16**(1):48-55. DOI:10.1016/j.ejpn.2011.10.003

[6] Graham HK, Rosenbaum P, Paneth N, et al. Cerebral palsy. Nature Reviews Disease Primers. 2016;**2**:15082. DOI:10.1038/nrdp.2015.82.

[7] Depositario-Cabacar DF, Zelleke TG. Treatment of epilepsy in children with developmental disabilities. Developmental Disabilities Research Reviews. 2010;**16**(3):239-247. DOI: 10.1002/ddrr.116

[8] Zelnik N, Konopnicki M, Bennett-Back O, et al. Risk factors for epilepsy in children with cerebral palsy. European Journal of Paediatric Neurology. 2010;14(1):67-72. DOI:10.1016/j.ejpn.2009.06.002

[9] Huo HL, Gu Q, Shi XY, et al. Analysis of related factors for children with cerebral palsy complicated by epilepsy. Medical Journal of Chinese People's Liberation Army. 2014;**26**(11):72-74, 78. DOI: 10.3969/j.issn.2095-140X.2014.11.018

[10] Zhang ZZ, Wu M. EEG characteristics of cerebral palsy combined with epilepsy. Journal of Clinical Medicine. 2006;**32**(5):350-351. DOI: 10.3969/j.issn.1673-1557.2006.05.018

[11] Wen XS, Deng FP, Zhang JM. Prognosis and clinic of epilepsy in children with cerebral palsy. Chinese Journal of Trauma and Disability Medicine. 2010;**18**(1):25-27. DOI: 10.3969/j.issn.1673-6567.2010.01.015

[12] Terra VC, Cysneiros RM, Schwartzman JS, et al. Mothers of children with cerebral palsy with or without epilepsy: a quality of life perspective. Disability and Rehabilitation. 2011;**33**(5):384-388. DOI:10.3109/09638281003611052

[13] Holmes GL. Cognitive impairment in epilepsy: the role of network abnormalities. Epileptic Disorders. 2015;**17**(2):101-116. DOI: 10.1684/epd.2015.0739

[14] Szpindel A, Myers KA, Ng P, Dorais M, Koclas L, Pigeon N, et al. Epilepsy in children with cerebral palsy: a data linkage study. Developmental Medicine and Child Neurology. 2022;**64**(2):259-265. DOI: 10.1111/dmcn.15028

[15] Carlsson M, Olsson I, Hagberg G, Beckung E. Behaviour in children with cerebral palsy with and without epilepsy. Developmental Medicine and Child Neurology. 2008;**50**(10):784-789. DOI: 10.1111/j.1469-8749.2008.03090.x

[16] McLellan A. Epilepsy-an additional risk factor for psychological problems in cerebral palsy. Developmental Medicine and Child Neurology. 2008;**50**(10):727. DOI: 10.1111/j.1469-8749.2008.03103.x

[17] Hanci F, Türay S, Dilek M, Kabakuş N. Epilepsy and drug-resistant epilepsy in children with cerebral palsy: a retrospective observational study. Epilepsy & Behavior. 2020;**112**:107357. DOI: 10.1016/j.yebeh.2020.107357

[18] El Tantawi NT, Abd Elmegid DS, Atef E. Seizure outcome and epilepsy patterns in patients with cerebral palsy. Seizure. 2019;**65**:166-171. DOI: 10.1016/j.seizure.2019.01.003

[19] Morgan C, Fahey M, Roy B, et al. Diagnosing cerebral palsy in full-term infants. Journal of Paediatrics and Child Health. 2018;**54**(10):1159-1164

[20] He X, Xu Y, Yang X. Precise diagnosis and treatment of spastic cerebral palsy. Zhongguo Xiu Fu Chong Jian Wai Ke Za Zhi. 2019;**33**(12):1584-1588

[21] Chin EM, Gwynn HE, Robinson S, et al. Principles of medical and surgical treatment of cerebral palsy. Neurologic Clinics. 2020;**38**(2):397-416

[22] Quitadamo P, Thapar N, Staiano A, et al. Gastrointestinal and nutritional problems in neurologically impaired children. European Journal of Paediatric Neurology. 2016;**20**(6):810-815

[23] Ivana T, Iva H. Evaluation and treatment of malnutrition and associated gastrointestinal complications in children with cerebral palsy. Pediatric Gastroenterology, Hepatology and Nutrition. 2019;**22**(2):122-131

[24] Huang C, Li Y, Feng X, et al. Distinct gut microbiota composition and functional category in children with cerebral palsy and epilepsy. Frontiers in Pediatrics. 2019;**7**:394

[25] Huang C, Peng Y, Li Y, et al. Changes in the gut microbiota in patients with cerebral palsy and epilepsy. Chinese Journal of Microecology. 2019;**31**(4):402-406

[26] Huang C, Li X, Wu L, et al. The effect of different dietary structure on gastrointestinal dysfunction in children with cerebral palsy and epilepsy based on gut microbiota. Brain and Development. 2021;**43**:192-199

[27] Vriesman MH, Rajindrajith S, IJN K, et al. Quality of life in children with functional constipation: a systematic review and meta-analysis. Journal of Pediatrics. 2019;**214**:141-150

[28] Boldyreva U, Streiner DL, Rosenbaum PL, Ronen GM. Quality of life in adolescents with epilepsy, cerebral palsy, and population norms. Developmental Medicine and Child Neurology. 2020;**62**(5):609-614. DOI: 10.1111/dmcn.14450

[29] Huang CF, Chu CN, Peng YP, Zhang N, Yang ZY, You J, Wei FX. Correlations between gastrointestinal and oral microbiota in children with cerebral palsy and epilepsy. Frontiers in Pediatrics 2022;10:988601. doi: 10.3389/fped.2022.988601

[30] Bensi C, Costacurta M, Docimo R. Oral health in children with cerebral palsy: a systematic review and meta-analysis. Special Care in Dentistry. 2020;**40**(5):401-411. DOI: 10.1111/scd.12506

[31] Akhter R, Hassan NM, Martin EF, Muhit M, Haque MR, et al. Risk factors for dental caries among children with cerebral palsy in a low-resource setting. Developmental Medicine and Child Neurology. 2017;**59**(5):538-543. DOI: 10.1111/dmcn.13359

[32] Xu Y, Jia YH, Chen L, et al. Metagenomic analysis of oral microbiome in young children aged 6-8 years living in a rural isolated Chinese Province. Oral Diseases. 2018;**24**(6):1115-1125

[33] Yang Z, Liu B. Advances on the studies on microecology of dental plaques in dental caries. International Journal of Stomatology. 2020;**47**(5):506-514

[34] Engevik MA, Danhof HA, Ruan W, Engevik AC, Chang-Graham AL, Engevik KA, et al. Fusobacterium nucleatum secretes outer membrane vesicles and promotes intestinal inflammation. mBio. 2021;**12**(2):e02706-e02720. DOI: 10.1128/mBio.02706-20

[35] Kitamoto S, Nagao-Kitamoto H, Hein R, Schmidt TM, Kamada N. The Bacterial Connection between the Oral Cavity and the Gut Diseases. Journal of Dental Research. 2020;**99**(9):1021-1029. DOI: 10.1177/0022034520924633

[36] Ferreira ACFM, Eveloff RJ, Freire M, Santos MTBR. The impact of oral-gut inflammation in cerebral palsy. Frontiers in Immunology. 2021;**12**:619262. DOI: 10.3389/fimmu.2021.619262

[37] Liu MX, Shi YH, Wu KB, Xie W, Ser HL, Jiang QZ, et al. From mouth to brain: distinct supragingival plaque microbiota composition in cerebral palsy children with caries. Frontiers in Cellular and Infection Microbiology. 2022;**12**:814473. DOI: 10.3389/fcimb.2022.814473

[38] Tanes C, Bittinger K, Gao Y, et al. Role of dietary fiber in the recovery of the human gut microbiome and its metabolome. Cell Host & Microbe. 2021;**29**(3):394-407.e5

[39] Camilleri M. Human intestinal barrier: effects of stressors, diet, prebiotics, and probiotics. Clinical and Translational Gastroenterology. 2021;**12**(1):e00308

[40] Choque Delgado GT, Tamashiro WMDSC. Role of prebiotics in regulation of microbiota and prevention of obesity. Food Research International. 2018;**113**:183-188

[41] Zhao X, Zhou J, Liang W, et al. Probiotics mixture reinforces barrier function to ameliorate necrotizing enterocolitis by regulating PXR-JNK pathway. Cell & Bioscience. 2021;**11**(1):20

[42] Huang CF, Lyu JL, Chu CN, Ge L, Peng YP, Yang ZY, et al. Dietary fiber and probiotics based on gut microbiota targeting for functional constipation in children with cerebral palsy. Frontiers in Pediatrics. 2022;**10**:1001789. DOI: 10.3389/fped.2022.1001789

Chapter 3

Perspective Chapter: Epilepsy and Pregnancy

Pavel Vlasov

Abstract

Currently, there are approximately 15 million women of childbearing age worldwide. A total of 0.3–0.4% of newborns are born to mothers with epilepsy, with nearly half a percent of these women experiencing ongoing seizures. This chapter addresses issues related to pregnancy preparation, the prognostic influence of seizure frequency, epilepsy type, and course on pregnancy outcomes, as well as potential risks associated with the condition for both the mother and the fetus. Summary data on latest recommendations for therapy adjustments and data on the pharmacokinetic changes of antiepileptic drugs during pregnancy are provided. The classification of antiepileptic drugs based on their teratogenic potential and their impact on child development and behavior is presented. Various approaches to managing pregnancy are discussed. Scenarios for managing pregnancy in cases of poorly controlled epilepsy and status epilepticus, as well as therapy adjustments in the postpartum period and measures for the safe care of newborns, are also considered.

Keywords: epilepsy, pregnancy, pregnant women with epilepsy, preparation for pregnancy, management of pregnancy, antiseizure drugs, postpartum, teratogenesis, major congenital malformations

1. Introduction

The management of pregnancy in women with epilepsy (WWE) is a relevant issue, considering the estimated global population of around 15 million women of reproductive age [1]. Statistical reports indicate that approximately 0.3–0.4% of newborns are born to mothers with epilepsy. Furthermore, the improved effectiveness of epilepsy therapy in the past two decades, with the use of new antiseizure drugs (ASDs), has led to a fourfold increase in pregnancies in women with epilepsy (WWE) [2]. The prevalence of active epilepsy among pregnant women is reported to be 0.33% [3], but other studies indicate a slightly higher rate of 0.49% [4]. Epileptic seizures rarely occur exclusively during pregnancy, which is known as gestational epilepsy.

2. Epilepsy and pregnancy

2.1 Seizure control during pregnancy

Several studies have indicated that the frequency of seizures during pregnancy remains unchanged [5]. However, when seizures have been in remission for 9 months or longer before conception, there is hope for their absence during pregnancy [6].

In a prospective observational multicenter cohort study conducted by Pennell et al. [5], the frequency of seizures during pregnancy and the first 6 weeks after delivery (n = 299) (observation period I) was compared with the frequency in the postpartum period (the subsequent 7.5 months after pregnancy) (period II). A control group (n = 93) consisted of nonpregnant women of similar age who were observed over an 18-month period. Patient demographics did not significantly differ between the groups. The primary outcome assessed was the percentage of women who experienced a higher frequency of seizures with impaired consciousness during period I compared to period II. Changes in ASD dosage were also evaluated in both groups. The results indicated that the frequency of seizures with impaired consciousness remained unchanged, worsened, or improved to a similar extent in both pregnant and nonpregnant women: unchanged frequency was reported in 63% of pregnant women and 65% of nonpregnant women, improvement in 14% and 11%, respectively, and worsening in 23% and 25%. In the pregnant group, 74% of the cases required a change in drug dosage or additional ASD prescription, while in the control group, dosage adjustments were necessary in only 31% of the cases [5].

According to the largest EURAP study (n = 3806 pregnancies), absence of seizures during pregnancy was observed in 66.6% of the cases. The rate increased to 73.6% for idiopathic generalized epilepsy (IGE) and decreased to 59.5% for focal epilepsy (FE) [7]. The average increase in ASD dosage from the first to the third trimester was 26% for lamotrigine, 5% for carbamazepine, 11% for phenobarbital, and 6% for valproate. The study reported 21 cases of epileptic status, 10 of which were convulsive, with no maternal mortality and only one case of stillbirth. The authors emphasize the need for more active adjustment of ASD dosages during pregnancy, particularly in cases of seizures occurring in the first trimester [7].

In a single-center study (114 pregnancies), Voinescu et al. [8] observed a significantly milder course of IGE and nonfrontal focal epilepsy during pregnancy, particularly when achieving seizure control for a 9-month period prior to pregnancy. A more detailed analysis of the results revealed that patients with frontal epilepsy experienced an increase in seizures during pregnancy (75%) when seizure control was not achieved before pregnancy, compared to an increase of 33% when seizure control was established prior to pregnancy. A similar disparity was observed in cases of focal epilepsy with different localizations; however, the percentage of seizure exacerbation was significantly lower (26% and 5%, respectively) [8].

In an observational cohort study conducted in Nigeria, a higher likelihood of seizures during pregnancy was observed in cases of structural focal epilepsy with posttraumatic (P = .013) and infectious etiology (P = .041). The authors also noted that the absence of seizures for less than 6 months before pregnancy had an unfavorable impact on pregnancy outcomes (P = .043) [3].

The review by Eadie [9] focuses on the analysis of seizure dynamics during pregnancy over the past 50 years. In the majority of studies, there was a predominant, albeit insignificant, trend toward worsened control of epileptic seizures during pregnancy. A detailed analysis of this worsening seizure control during pregnancy

Author	Number of pregnant WWE (n)	Number of women (n)	Seizure reduction rate (%)	Seizure exacerbation rate (%)
Battino et al. 2013 [7]	3806	3451	12%	15.8%
Reisinger et al. 2013 [10]	115	95	17.4%	38.3%
Cagnetti et al. 2014 [11]		272	17.5%	23.4%
La Neve et al. 2015 [12]	56		8%	19%
Shahla et al. 2018 [13]		94	25.5%	28.7%
Pennell et al. 2020 [5]		351	14%	23%
Voinescu et al. 2022 [8]	114	99		21.1% for FE 5.3% for IGE

WWE—women with epilepsy; FE—focal epilepsy; IGE—idiopathic generalized epilepsy.

Table 1.
Seizure dynamics during pregnancy according to Eadie (2021) [9] with supplemental data.

identified several contributing factors, including the use of ASDs with lower teratogenic potential but less stable pharmacokinetics during pregnancy, noncompliance, the influence of steroid sex hormones on the estrogen/progesterone ratio, a more unfavorable course of focal epilepsy compared to generalized epilepsy, remission of seizures for less than 9–12 months before conception, and the use of monotherapy or polytherapy (polytherapy likely indicating pharmacoresistant disease) [9]. Additionally, negative influences on the course of epilepsy during pregnancy include nonadherence to a sleep-wake schedule (particularly in cases of generalized epilepsy), vomiting during pregnancy, anxiety, and depression [2].

As indicated in the **Table 1**, nearly all publications in the last 10 years report a predominance (sometimes minor) of increased seizure frequency during pregnancy compared to seizure reduction [9].

A limited number of studies have examined the dynamics of epilepsy during pregnancy in the absence of ASD therapy. The main conclusion drawn from observations of patients who refused to take ASDs during the first trimester or throughout their pregnancy is that their seizure frequency increased [14].

There are differing opinions regarding the influence of a previous pregnancy on the course of a current one. According to one viewpoint, an unfavorable course of a previous pregnancy increases the likelihood of decompensation in subsequent pregnancies. However, our experience suggests that such prediction is not possible [2].

To summarize the key points on Seizure control during pregnancy:

1. Achieving seizure control for 9 months before pregnancy is associated with a high likelihood of its maintaining during pregnancy [6].

2. The largest study (EURAP) reported a probability of seizure absence during pregnancy of 59.5% for focal epilepsy, 73.6% for IGE, and an average of 66.6% [7].

3. Frontal lobe epilepsy is more likely to worsen during pregnancy compared to other types of focal epilepsy [8].

4. Among focal epilepsies, there is a higher likelihood of increased seizures during pregnancy in cases of structural focal epilepsy (due to trauma or encephalitis) [3].

5. Status epilepsticus occurs during pregnancy in 0.55% of cases [7].

6. "Old" ASDs such as phenobarbital, valproate, and carbamazepine were found to be more effective in treating focal and generalized epilepsy during pregnancy [7]. However, valproate (and possibly phenobarbital according to some data) is not recommended for use during pregnancy due to its high teratogenic potential in terms of structural and cognitive effects [15].

7. Factors such as compliance, avoidance of smoking and alcohol and drug use, sufficient sleep (especially in the case of IGE), identification and timely therapy of anxiety/depression, and repeated administration of ASDs in case of vomiting during epilepsy shortly after ASD administration play an important role in maintaining stable seizure control during pregnancy [2].

2.2 Epileptic seizures: risk for mother and fetus

The main objective of using ASDs is to prevent seizure occurrence during pregnancy, as they have unfavorable effects on both the mother and the fetus/child. Generalized tonic-clonic seizures and focal seizures to bilateral tonic-clonic seizures have the most harmful impact on the mother, including the possibility of traumatic brain injury, limb injury, spinal cord injuries, blunt abdominal trauma, hypoxia, lactic acidosis, etc. [2]. Sudden unexpected death in epilepsy (SUDEP) is also a concern [16]. These seizures can also have adverse effects on the fetus, such as asphyxia, hypoxia, and trauma [15]. All other seizures have minimal impact unless they are associated with falls of pregnant WWE [2]. Focal seizures with impaired consciousness have been described to cause a short-term fetal distress syndrome characterized by a decrease in fetal heart rate to 3.5 min [17].

The presence of seizures during pregnancy, regardless of classification, was reported to lead to decreased size and weight of the newborn as well as premature birth [18].

Currently, there is no evidence of a direct link between seizures and the occurrence of major congenital malformations (MCM) in the fetus [15]. However, certain conditions can increase the likelihood of MCM, such as prolonged generalized tonic-clonic seizures or status epilepticus, which can result in severe hypoxia and acidosis. Depending on the gestational age at which the seizure occurred, pregnancy outcomes vary. If there is a significant loss of germinal material miscarriage occurs. In case of complete regeneration of germinal material, structural defects do not develop. During the period of histogenesis and organogenesis, the development of MCM is possible, while in the second and third trimesters, the development of minor anomalies, developmental delays, and adverse cognitive and behavioral consequences may occur. Nevertheless, prospective studies have not yet confirmed the influence of generalized tonic-clonic seizures on the development of the nervous system [19, 20].

2.2.1 Pharmacokinetics of ASD during pregnancy

Significant changes in the pharmacokinetics of ASDs occur during pregnancy, starting from the early stages, including alterations in absorption, increased distribution volume, enhanced renal excretion, and induction of hepatic metabolism. **Table 2** presents summarized data on predicting ASD concentrations during pregnancy with an unchanged daily dose.

ASD	Decrease in serum concentration	Decrease in serum free (unbound) concentration	Recommendations to perform therapeutic drug monitoring, if available
Phenobarbital	Up to 55%	Up to 50%	Yes
Phenytoin	60–70%	20–40%	Yes, free concentration
Carbamazepine	0–12%	None	Optional
Valproate	Up to 23%	None	Optional, free concentration if done
Oxcarbazepine monohydroxy-derivative (MHD)	36–62%	N/A	Yes
Lamotrigine	0.77 of population: 69% decrease 0.23 of population: 17% decrease	N/A	Yes
Topiramate	Up to 30%	N/A	Yes
Levetiracetam	40–60%, with maximal decrease reached in first trimester	N/A	Yes
Zonisamide	Up to 35%; data is limited	N/A	Yes

N/A: not applicable.

Table 2.
Summary data on prediction of individual ASD concentrations during pregnancy with unchanged daily dose of ASD (AED—antiepileptic drug) daily dose according to Tomson et al. [15] with modifications.

As indicated in **Table 2**, the most unstable pharmacokinetics during pregnancy are observed when using phenobarbital (PHB), phenytoin (PHT), oxcarbazepine (OXC), lamotrigine (LTG), levetiracetam (LEV), ZNS, gababentin (GBP). Therefore, during pregnancy, the concentration of these ASDs should be monitored. In several studies by Harden et al. [6], Reisinger et al. [10], and Voinescu et al. [21], a critical decrease in ASD concentration was identified, which constituted 65% of the concentration before pregnancy [6, 10, 21]. Accordingly, a decrease in the concentration by just 35% can lead to an increase in epileptic seizures. If monitoring concentration is not possible, it is necessary to increase the daily dose of ASDs with variable pharmacokinetics by 30–50% in advance, especially in cases of unstable disease progression, short-term medication remission, initial difficulty in selecting therapy, structural focal epilepsy, history of generalized tonic-clonic seizures or focal seizures with impaired awareness, and with a minimal daily dose of ASDs [22].

2.2.2 The impact of ASDs on fetal growth and development

The impact of ASDs on fetal growth and development has been extensively studied using data from national registries and population-based studies, including those conducted in Australia, Denmark, Finland, Norway, Russia [23], EURAP, NAAPR, NEAD, Sweden, and the UK and Ireland Epilepsy and Pregnancy Registers. The findings suggest that the use of polytherapy during pregnancy, as well as monotherapy with Primidone, Phenobarbital, carbamazepine (CBZ), valproic acid (VPA), and newer ASDs such as topiramate (TPM) and zonisamide (ZNS), may be associated with varying degrees of intrauterine growth restriction, with TPM having the greatest negative impact [15]. The prospective NEAD study revealed an increased incidence of microcephaly with the use of VPA and CBZ during pregnancy, although by the age of 2 years, the child's head size was not significantly different from population norms (the measures were equalized) [24].

2.2.3 Teratogenesis

ASDs have been classified into categories based on their teratogenic potential, with LTG and LEV having minimal potential, pregabalin and TPM having moderate potential, and VPA having the highest potential (**Table 3**) [15]. However, the results of a nationwide cohort study conducted in France over a period of more than 4 years, involving all pregnancies ≥20 weeks (n = 1,886,825), did not show significant associations with major congenital malformations (MCM) for LTG, LEV, OXC, and CBZ [29]. For drugs with high and moderate risks of congenital malformations, there is a direct correlation between the increase in daily dosage and the frequency of MCM, particularly for VPA [15]. Furthermore, a specific organ-specificity of congenital malformation development has been demonstrated: for VPA, eight associations were identified, including spina bifida, four cardiovascular variants, facial anomalies, anorectal anomalies, and hypospadias. In the case of TPM, cleft palate and cleft lip were observed, while cardiac malformations were associated with the use of barbiturates (**Table 4**).

In recent years, the perspective on the use of bi- or polytherapy has shifted, focusing on the specific drugs involved rather than the fact of polytherapy itself. Data from the Australian registry indicate that any combination of ASDs with VPA and TPM is not recommended, whereas combining ASDs with LTG and LEV does not significantly increase the risk [28]. However, if the use of VPA and TPM during pregnancy cannot be avoided, it is advised to administer them at the minimum effective doses necessary to control generalized tonic-clonic seizures and focal to bilateral tonic-clonic seizures.

2.2.4 Fetal anticonvulsant syndrome

Fetal anticonvulsant syndrome, also known as fetal embryopathy or fetal anticonvulsant (primidone, hydantoin, phenobarbital, valproate, carbamazepine)

ASD	**The rate of congenital malformations development**			
	EURAP [25]	**NAAPR [26]**	**UK and Ireland [27]**	**Australian [28]**
Carbamazepine	5.5%	3.0%	2.6%	5.5%
Valproic acid	10.3%	9.3%	6.7%	13.8%
Phenobarbital	6.5%	5.5%		
Topiramate	3.9%	4.2%	4.3%	2.4%
Lamotrigine	2.9%	2.0%	2.3%	4.6%
Levetiracetam	2.8%	2.4%	0.7%	2.4%
Phenytoin	6.4%	2.9%	3.7%	
Oxcarbazepine	3.0%	2.2%		

Table 3.
Prevalence of major congenital malformations with monotherapy based on data from 4 prospective registries according to Tomson et al. [15] with supplemental information.

ASD	Malformation type	Odds Ratio [95% confidence interval]
Topiramate	Cleft lip or cleft palate	6.8 [1.4–20.0]
Barbiturates	Congenital Heart Defects	10.5 [1.3–39.3]
Valproate	Spina bifida	19.4 [8.6–43.5]
	Ventricular septal defect	4.0 [2.1–7.8]
	Patent foramen ovale	9.0 [5.4–15.0]
	Pulmonary atresia	27.8 [3.3–102.5]
	Hypoplastic left heart syndrome	19.6 [2.4–71.7]
	Cleft palate	5.4 [1.1–15.8]
	Anorectal atresia	11.7 [2.4–34.4]
	Hypospadias	4.8 [2.4–9.8]

Table 4.
ASDs and the associated MCMs according to Blotière et al. [29].

syndrome, is a condition that occurs with the use of ASDs during pregnancy. It is characterized by minor structural abnormalities in the fetus that do not typically require treatment. Although this aspect of ASD use has received limited attention in recent scientific literature, information on this issue can be obtained from the Genetic and Rare Disease (GARD) website (https://rarediseases.info.nih.gov/diseases/6435/fetal-hydantoin-syndrome).

2.2.5 The impact of ASDs on child development and behavior

In addition to structural teratogenesis, there is also a phenomenon known as "cognitive teratogenesis."

VPA takes precedence in terms of cognitive, as well as structural teratogenesis. The use of valproate during pregnancy in WWE is associated with a significant dose-dependent risk of cognitive impairments and developmental disorders of the nervous system in the child, as well as an increased occurrence of autistic spectrum disorders. In utero exposure to VPA has been correlated with developmental problems in infancy [30], decreased IQ and cognitive function impairments during childhood [31], and adolescence [32]. Prenatal exposure to VPA is also linked to a higher risk of developing autistic spectrum disorders, attention deficit hyperactivity disorder, and other behavioral problems [33]. There is a clear dose-dependent relationship, with even low doses of VPA (less than 400 mg/day) associated with decreased verbal IQ and increased need for educational assistance [19, 20, 34].

Research on the intrauterine effects of CBZ suggests that this drug does not cause serious neurobehavioral disorders. However, there are risks associated with reduced verbal reasoning skills [20, 35], as well as slightly poorer performance in mathematics compared to the control group, although the difference was not significant [36]. Previous data on the development of autism spectrum disorders were not confirmed in subsequent national cohort studies, large observational studies, or studies based on parents' assessments of autistic behavior symptoms in children [33].

Limited information is available regarding the effects of phenytoin monotherapy on cognitive and behavioral functions and socialization due to small sample sizes.

However, some studies have shown that children exposed to phenytoin have higher IQs compared to children exposed to VPA, and their IQs are comparable to those on CBZ and LTG monotherapy [19, 34].

The best outcomes have been observed in children born to mothers who received LTG during pregnancy, with their IQs being comparable to those of children in the control group [20]. Children exposed to intrauterine LTG exposure have shown better results in early development and school periods compared to children whose mothers received VPA [19]. Furthermore, no higher risk of autism spectrum disorders has been found in this group [37].

Limited information is available regarding the effects of LEV, TPM, and other ASDs on cognitive performance and behavior in later childhood [15]. In conclusion, regarding the intrauterine effects of ASDs on children of WWE, it is important to note the lack of reliable data for most currently prescribed ASDs. Further studies on this issue are required, and the absence of evidence of harm should not be interpreted as evidence of the safety of any given ASD. When preparing for pregnancy, patients should discuss the known risk and benefit information for individual ASDs that is available at the time.

To summarize the key points on epilepsy and pregnancy:

1. Achieving seizure control for 9 months prior to pregnancy increases the likelihood of maintaining this control during pregnancy. Generalized tonic-clonic and focal to bilateral tonic-clonic seizures have the most unfavorable impact on both the mother and fetus.

2. IGE has a 10% higher rate of remission maintenance during pregnancy compared to FE. Structural FE and, in particular, frontal lobe epilepsy have a higher likelihood of seizure aggravation during pregnancy. Status epilepticus occurs in 0.5% of pregnant WWE.

3. "Old" ASDs such as phenobarbital, valproate, and carbamazepine have shown higher effectiveness in focal and generalized epilepsy during pregnancy. However, valproate is not recommended due to its high teratogenic potential.

4. Different ASDs have varying levels of teratogenic potential. Lamotrigine, levetiracetam, oxcarbazepine, and carbamazepine are considered to have minimal teratogenic potential, while topiramate and valproate have moderate to maximum teratogenic potential.

5. Changes in pharmacokinetics of ASDs during pregnancy necessitate monitoring and adjustment of daily dosage. Monitoring ASD serum concentrations is important, as some drugs (lamotrigine, levetiracetam, oxcarbazepine, phenobarbital, phenytoin, topiramate, and zonisamide) may exhibit significant increases or decreases of ASD elimination during pregnancy, affecting seizure control. A decrease in serum concentrations greater than 35% of optimal pre-pregnancy concentrations is associated with an increased risk of impaired seizure control.

6. The impact on pregnancy is attributed to the ASDs included in the dual therapy regimen, rather than the dual therapy itself. If the use of valproate and topiramate is necessary during pregnancy, minimal doses that control generalized tonic-clonic and focal to bilateral tonic-clonic seizures should be administered.

7. Factors such as compliance, avoidance of smoking, alcohol and drug use, sufficient sleep (especially for IGE), identification and timely treatment of anxiety/depression, and repeated intake of ASDs in case of vomiting shortly after administration all contribute to maintaining a stable condition during pregnancy.

3. Management of pregnancy in epilepsy

3.1 Therapy

The protocols for treatment of pregnant WWE are based on expert opinions and consensuses and incorporate evidence-based practices. Nowadays, epilepsy treatment utilizes a variety of ASDs. The treatment approach emphasizes adherence to lifestyle recommendations, such as the avoidance of sleep deprivation, alcohol consumption, and reflex stimuli in reflex epilepsy. Additionally, it involves strict adherence to the prescribed medication regimen and use of the appropriate dosages prescribed by an epileptologist. Monotherapy with a single ASD at the minimum effective daily dose is the preferred approach. Combination therapy with two or, in rare cases, three ASDs that exhibit synergistic pharmacodynamics and pharmacokinetics may be considered if monotherapy proves ineffective [22].

3.1.1 Drug therapy

The latest recommendations from the working group on providing assistance to pregnant WWE suggest that LTG, LEV, OXC, and, to a lesser extent, CBZ are not significantly associated with the development of congenital malformations in fetus [15]. While, the use of VPA and phenobarbital in women of childbearing age is generally discouraged [38]. If discontinuation of these drugs is not possible during preparation for pregnancy, it is recommended to use two ASDs at a minimal dose of VPA, with LTG, LEV, OXC, or CBZ serving as potential additional options.

3.1.2 Role of folic acid

For several decades, the administration of folic acid to patients with epilepsy before conception and during pregnancy has been considered essential. Studies have shown that folate supplementation reduces the incidence of congenital heart defects [39], lowers the risk of autistic spectrum disorders [40], and contributes to increased IQ in children born to mothers with epilepsy who take ASDs [19]. Population studies have also indicated a positive effect of folic acid on the development of the nervous system, behavior, verbal abilities [41], although further research is needed to gain additional evidence.

The recommended daily dose of folic acid varies significantly, ranging from 0.4 mg/day [42] to 5 mg/day [15]. Higher doses of folate, exceeding 0.4 mg/day, are recommended in cases where a family history of malformations is identified. However, it is important to note that the administration of increased doses of folic acid has been associated with an increased risk of oncological diseases, cognitive disorders, and cleft palate [43]. Therefore, ongoing research in this area is necessary. In our work, we recommend regular intake of folic acid at a dose of 3 mg for 1–2 months before conception and during the first 12 weeks of pregnancy [22]. However, obstetricians often recommend folate intake of at least 0.4 mg daily for women of childbearing age due to the high risk of unplanned pregnancies.

3.2 Preparation for pregnancy

Preparation for pregnancy begins during the puberty, when discussions about pregnancy and contraception are initiated with the patient and her relatives, including her mother and grandmother. Since epilepsy requires constant use of ASDs, the primary goal for a neurologist or an epileptologist is to achieve a seizure remission for at least 9 months prior to planned pregnancy using monotherapy with the minimum effective dosage of ASDs. Studies suggest that a period without seizures for 6 months is generally sufficient, but further research is needed to gather more data [2]. The need for continuous use of ASDs is justified by the fact that the risks associated with generalized seizures are greater for the patient and her child than the potential risks of continuous ASD usage [2, 15, 22, 23]. In preparation for pregnancy, in addition to selecting appropriate ASDs, a general physical examination is mandatory to exclude nonneurological diseases, particularly anemia, and assess the functional state of parenchymal organs involved in ASDs metabolism and elimination, namely the liver and kidneys.

The algorithm for preparing for pregnancy and managing pregnant WWE is presented in **Figure 1**. For ASDs such as LEV, LTG, OXC, ZNS, PHB, PHT, and benzodiazepines, it is important to consider the decrease in drug concentration due to increased renal blood flow starting from the end of the first trimester. Thus, physicians should be aware of the baseline concentration of ASD with variable pharmacokinetics before pregnancy and strive to maintain that baseline level throughout pregnancy. LTG exhibits the most significant changes in pharmacokinetics, with potential for threefold decrease in serum concentration, necessitating an increase in the daily dosage of the drug. The International League Against Epilepsy recommends monitoring these ASDs every 4 weeks, considering a clinically significant decrease in concentration by at least one-third of the original level. Therefore, if it is not possible to measure the ASD concentration during pregnancy, a 30–50% increase in the daily dosage is recommended at the end of the first trimester for patients on a minimal dose of ASDs with variable pharmacokinetics (LTG, LEV, OXC, ZNS, PHB, PHT), if these patients experience generalized tonic-clonic seizures or other seizure types associated with falls. The question of increasing the daily dosage should also be considered in cases of short-term, unstable remission in pregnant WWE with significant structural brain changes and in cases of polytherapy involving ASDs with variable pharmacokinetics [15].

3.3 Assisted reproductive technologies

During in vitro fertilization with high doses of estrogens, it is important to consider the possible recurrence of epileptic seizures, as estrogens have pro-epileptic effects unlike progesterone. Furthermore, the use of female steroid sex hormones can significantly affect the pharmacokinetics of LTG, a commonly used antiepileptic drug, leading to a reduction in its blood levels by 2 or more times. Therefore, in cases of long-lasting, persistent drug-induced clinical remission, it is recommended to continue regular use of antiepileptic drugs and maintain a consistent sleep-wake cycle. Before performing ovarian stimulation procedures in patients with

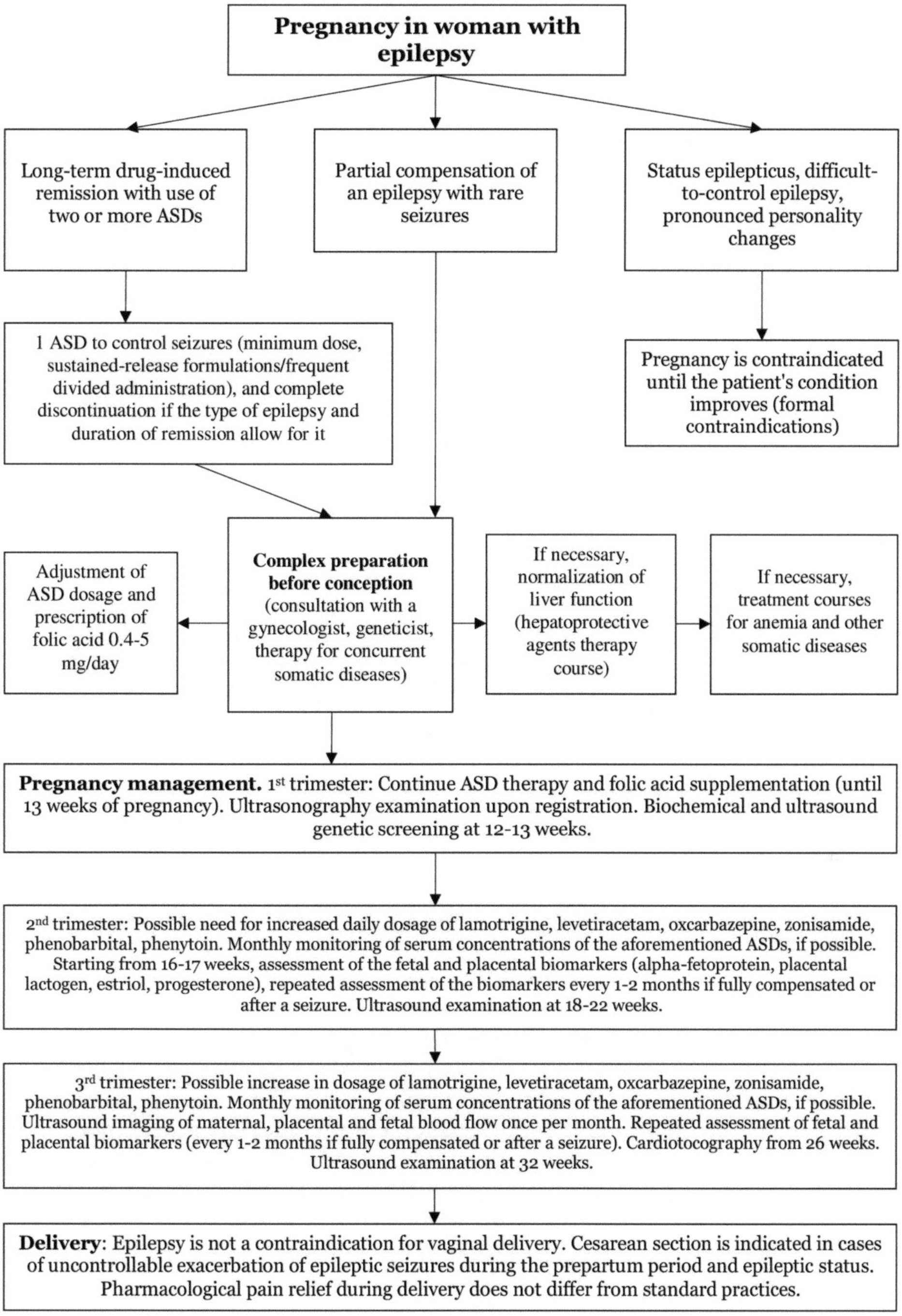

Figure 1.
Algorithm for preparing for pregnancy, management of pregnancy and delivery in patients with epilepsy [22].

insufficiently compensated primary disease state, it is desirable to assess the blood levels of antiepileptic drugs both initially and during sex hormone administration [22]. If the concentration of antiepileptic drugs is reduced by one-third, it is recommended to increase the daily dose by 30–50%. If it is not possible to determine the concentration of LTG, its dosage should be increased by 50% before undergoing in vitro fertilization.

3.4 Management of pregnancy in epilepsy

There are formal contraindications to pregnancy, which include difficult-to-control epilepsy with frequent epileptic seizures accompanied by falls, generalized tonic-clonic or focal to bilateral tonic-clonic seizures, status epilepticus, and marked personality changes posing a threat to the health and life of both the mother and the fetus [2, 22]. These contraindications are considered formal because if a woman decides to become pregnant, neurologists and obstetricians are obligated to use all possible means to preserve the pregnancy.

Given the certain risk of developing MCM, consultation with a geneticist is mandatory. Invasive methods of genetic testing may be performed based on specific indications.

In cases of compensated epilepsy with seizure remission, regular visits to the neurologist are required every 2 months, while visits to the obstetrician-gynecologist should follow standard guidelines. For patients experiencing focal seizures, more frequent visits to the neurologist every month are recommended, with visits to the obstetrician-gynecologist occurring every 2–3 weeks. Patients and their relatives should be strongly advised to consult an epileptologist if seizures occur more frequently. Increased or exacerbated seizures may be caused by sleep deprivation, concurrent diseases, medication regimen violations, and others. Epilepsy itself is not an indication for pregnant women to receive inpatient treatment in a specialized neurological department.

The determination of ASD concentrations is performed every 2 months or less frequently during compensated epilepsy, and in cases of observed seizures, once a month or at every visit to the neurologist during pregnancy. During the first trimester of pregnancy, it is necessary to investigate the concentrations of ASDs with variable pharmacokinetics, including LTG, LEV, OXC, TPM, felbamate, and ZNS. It is known that clearance increases at the end of the first trimester due to increased renal blood flow, which can subsequently lead to decreased ASD concentrations. In the case of LTG, increase in clearance, glucuronidation and conjugation, can collectively reduce its concentration by up to three times [44, 45].

The concentrations of hormones of the fetoplacental complex (placental lactogen, progesterone, estriol, cortisol) and alpha-fetoprotein should be studied starting from the end of the first trimester of pregnancy and subsequently no less than once a month. Dynamic ultrasound examination of the fetus should be performed when the pregnant woman is registered, at 19–21 weeks (to exclude fetal developmental anomalies), and at 30–31 weeks. Starting from the 20th week of pregnancy, it is advisable to perform Doppler assessment of blood flow in the umbilical artery, aorta, and middle cerebral artery of the fetus during ultrasound examination, considering the high risk of developing placental insufficiency. When performing ultrasound associations of different congenital malformations, anomalies with certain ASDs should be taken into account.

From the 26th week of pregnancy, the use of cardiotocography is recommended to provide an objective assessment of uterine motility and fetal condition.

Diagnosis and treatment of fetal growth restriction and placental dysfunction should follow standard protocols. In patients with controlled epilepsy, i.e. in a state of medical (and non-medical) remission, there are no peculiarities in prenatal preparation [22].

3.5 Status epilepticus

The treatment of generalized tonic-clonic seizures and focal to bilateral tonic-clonic seizures should follow the latest recommendations of 2020 [46]. Indications for Cesarean section include status epilepticus in the prepartum period. Status epilepticus of focal seizures without or with impaired consciousness and absence of status epilepticus does not serve as indications for pregnancy termination or C-section. All decisions regarding the treatment strategy and the prolongation of pregnancy during the status epilepticus should be made by a multidisciplinary team consisting of an obstetrician, neurologist, and anesthesiologist (perinatologist). Therefore, C-section is performed in all cases based on obstetric indications, except for status epilepticus in the prepartum period.

3.6 Delivery, pain relief, and pregnancy outcomes

Epilepsy is not a contraindication for vaginal delivery. Along with generally accepted obstetric indications, status epilepticus and uncontrolled increase in frequency of epileptic seizures in the prepartum period are grounds for performing a cesarean section [22].

Pharmacological intervention in labor and delivery and pain relief in epilepsy do not differ from the usual approach. Contraindications for epidural anesthesia are very rare, particularly in cases of impaired cerebrospinal fluid circulation due to acute cerebral and/or spinal pathology in the past.

Currently, there is insufficient data confirming or refuting the necessity of prescribing Vitamin K to a newborn during the early postpartum period when using ASDs with the aim to stimulate the cytochrome C450 enzymes [42]. Previous studies indicate a balance in the hemostasis system of newborns regardless of the ASDs used [47].

3.7 Postpartum management

Due to the risk of epileptic seizures during the postpartum period, the regular intake of prescribed ASD and sufficient rest are strongly recommended [2, 15].

The decrease in concentration of ASD required for seizure control after delivery can lead to the overdose, especially in cases of increased daily doses during pregnancy, potentially resulting in intoxication. There are reported cases of ASD overdose in the early postpartum period, with symptoms such as drowsiness, nystagmus, and ataxia in women, requiring a reduction in daily dosage and immediate monitoring of drug concentrations. The overdose of ASDs is attributed to a relative increase in concentration due to a mother weight decrease, blood loss during delivery, changes in ASD absorption, and other factors. Generally, returning to the daily dosage used before pregnancy is sufficient in the postpartum period, especially in cases when the daily dose of ASD was increased during pregnancy. According to the recommendations of Tomson et al. [1, 15], the normalization of lamotrigine pharmacokinetics occurs over the course of 3 weeks in the postpartum period [15]. However, there have been no observed signs of ASD overdose in the postpartum period in our practice [22].

If seizures persist or there is a risk of their occurrence or recurrence, it is recommended to have a relative constantly present with the mother. Seizures that can result in falls and harm the baby include generalized tonic-clonic, focal to bilateral tonic-clonic, atonic, myoclonic, and myoclonic-tonic-clonic seizures. Any epileptic seizure with impairment of consciousness also poses a danger to the baby. In all these situations, the newborn care, including bathing, diapering, and carrying, should be done with constant assistance from relatives [22].

There is no justification for discontinuing breastfeeding of a newborn since, during pregnancy the fetus is usually exposed to higher concentrations of ASDs than a newborn receiving ASD through a breast milk [15]. Breastfeeding should be done in a lying position to prevent injury in case a seizure occurs.

To summarize the key points on Management of Pregnancy in Epilepsy:

1. For women with epilepsy, treatment with ASD during pregnancy is usually necessary.

2. The primary treatment goal during preparation for pregnancy and management of pregnant WWE is to prevent generalized tonic-clonic seizures and focal to bilateral tonic-clonic seizures. Focal and generalized nonconvulsive seizures are generally considered harmless in terms of their impact on pregnancy and fetal development.

3. Patients should prepare for pregnancy. The main objective of such preparation is to achieve a drug-induced remission of generalized seizures, preferably using the lowest effective daily dose of a single medication.

4. The choice of antiseizure drug depends on achieving drug-induced remission. No antiepileptic drug is completely safe in terms of teratogenic effects. Lamotrigine, levetiracetam, oxcarbazepine, and to a lesser extent, carbamazepine, are currently believed to have the lowest teratogenic potential. If the patient's condition allows, it is preferable to avoid antiepileptic medication during pregnancy.

5. The management of pregnancy in women with epilepsy requires a comprehensive multidisciplinary approach involving a neurologist-epileptologist, obstetrician, and geneticist.

6. Indications for cesarean section are uncontrolled epilepsy in the prenatal period and status epilepticus.

7. In the prenatal period, adherence to general lifestyle recommendations and treatment regimens is crucial. In most cases, natural breastfeeding is practiced if the infant's condition allows it.

4. Conclusion

Research on the topic of "Epilepsy and Pregnancy" is an ongoing process, but many aspects still need to be studied. The analysis of publications is challenging due to multiple limitations such as small sample sizes, insufficient study quality, ethical constraints on conducting placebo-controlled studies, and other factors. Therefore, the main recommendations for managing epilepsy in pregnancy are based on expert opinions rather than strictly high-level evidence-based research. Nevertheless, significant progress has been made in recent years. Notably, the publication of "Management of epilepsy in pregnancy: a report from the International League Against Epilepsy Task Force on Women and Pregnancy" [15] provides valuable insights into the main issues, directions for further research, and recommendations for preparing and managing pregnancy in patients with epilepsy. A condensed version of the article with key positions was also published [1]. In 2020, the same group of researchers conducted a global survey of International League Against Epilepsy (ILAE) national chapters to assess the current state of the problem worldwide. The survey revealed that many countries still rely on outdated or overly general guidelines, while information on the topic is continuously evolving. The working group plans to collaborate with the ILAE Wikipedia team to create a series of pages containing updated recommendations for pregnancy in women with epilepsy and their care, ensuring that the latest information becomes available [48].

Conflict of interest

The authors declare no conflict of interest.

Author details

Pavel Vlasov
Moscow State University of Medicine and Dentistry named after A.I. Evdokimov, Moscow, Russia

*Address all correspondence to: vpn_neuro@mail.ru

References

[1] Tomson T, Battino D, Bromley R, Kochen S, Meador K, Pennel P, et al. Management of epilepsy in pregnancy: A report from the international league against epilepsy task force on women and pregnancy. Epilepsia. 2019;**00**:1-3. DOI: 10.1111/epi.16395

[2] Karlov VA, Vlasov PN, Petrukhin VA, Zhidkova IA, Adamyan LV. Chapter 32.3 epilepsy and pregnancy. In: Karlov VA, editor. Epilepsy in Children and Adults, Women, and Men: A Guide for Physicians. 2nd ed. Moscow: BINOM Publishing House; 2019. pp. 672-691

[3] Watila MM, Beida O, Kwari S, et al. Seizure occurrence, pregnancy outcome among women with active convulsive epilepsy: One year prospective study. Seizure. 2015;**26**:7-11. DOI: 10.1016/j.seizure.2015.01.007

[4] De Lima LM, Toporcov TN, Dal Pai J, Claudio da Silva J. Socio-demographic profiles and obstetrics outcomes of pregnant women with epilepsy in a vulnerability state, Brazil. PLoS One. 2022;**17**(7):e0271328. DOI: 10.1371/journal.pone.0271328

[5] Pennell PB, French JA, May RC, et al. Changes in seizure frequency and antiepileptic therapy during pregnancy. The New England Journal of Medicine. 2020;**383**(26):2547-2556. DOI: 10.1056/NEJMoa2008663

[6] Harden CL, Hopp J, Ting TY, et al. Management issues for women with epilepsy—Focus on pregnancy (an evidence-based review): I. Obstetrical complications and change in seizure frequency: Report of the quality standards subcommittee and therapeutics and technology assessment Subcommittee of the American Academy of neurology and the American Epilepsy Society. Epilepsia. 2009;**50**:1229-1236. DOI: 10.1111/j.1528-1167.2009.02128.x

[7] Battino D, Tomson T, Bonizzoni E, et al. Seizure control and treatment changes in pregnancy: Observations from the EURAP epilepsy pregnancy registry. Epilepsia. 2013;**54**(9):1621-1627

[8] Voinescu PE, Ehlert AN, Bay CP, Allien S, Pennell PB. Variations in seizure frequency during pregnancy and postpartum by epilepsy type. Neurology. 2022;**98**:e802-e807. DOI: 10.1212/WNL.0000000000013056

[9] Eadie MJ. Pregnancy and the control of epileptic seizures: A review. Neurology and Therapy. 2021;**10**(2):455-468. DOI: 10.1007/s40120-021-00252-5

[10] Reisinger TL, Newman M, Loring DW, Pennell PB, Meador KJ. Antiepileptic drug clearance and seizure frequency during pregnancy in women with epilepsy. Epilepsy & Behavior. 2013;**29**(1):13-18. DOI: 10.1016/j.yebeh.2013.06.026

[11] Cagnetti C, Lattanzi S, Foschi N, Provinciali L, Silvestrini M. Seizure course during pregnancy in catamenial epilepsy. Neurology. 2014;**83**:339-344. DOI: 10.1212/WNL.0000000000000619

[12] La Neve A, Boero G, Francavilla T, Plantamura M, De Agazio G, Specchio LM. Prospective, case-control study on the effect of pregnancy on seizure frequency in women with epilepsy. Neurological Sciences. 2015;**36**:79-83. DOI: 10.1007/s10072-014-1908-0

[13] Shahla M, Hijran B, Sharif M. The course of epilepsy and seizure control

in pregnant women. Acta Neurologica Belgica. 2018;**118**:459-464. DOI: 10.1007/s13760-018-0974-0

[14] Vajda FJ, O'Brien TJ, Lander CM, Graham J, Eadie MJ. Does pregnancy per se make epilepsy worse? Acta Neurologica Scandinavica. 2016;**133**:380-383. DOI: 10.1111/ane.12479

[15] Tomson T, Battino D, Bromley R, Kochen S, Meador K, Pennell P, et al. Management of epilepsy in pregnancy: A report from the international league against epilepsy task force on women and pregnancy. Epileptic Disorders. 2019;**21**(6):497-517. DOI: 10.1684/epd.2019.1105

[16] Edey S, Moran N, Nashef L. SUDEP and epilepsy-related mortality in pregnancy. Epilepsia. 2014;**55**(7):e72-e74. DOI: 10.1111/epi.12621

[17] Sahoo S, Klein P. Maternal complex partial seizure associated with fetal distress. Archives of Neurology. 2005;**62**(8):1304-1305. DOI: 10.1001/archneur.62.8.1304

[18] Chen YH, Chiou HY, Lin HC, Lin HL. Affect of seizures during gestation on pregnancy outcomes in women with epilepsy. Archives of Neurology. 2009;**66**:979-984. DOI: 10.1001/archneurol.2009.142

[19] Meador KJ, Baker GA, Browning N, et al. Fetal antiepileptic drug exposure and cognitive outcomes at age 6 years (NEAD study): A prospective observational study. Lancet Neurology. 2013;**12**(3):244-252. DOI: 10.1016/S1474-4422(12)70323-X

[20] Baker GA, Bromley RL, Briggs M, et al. IQ at 6 years after in utero exposure to antiepileptic drugs: A controlled cohort study. Neurology. 2015;**84**(4):382-390. DOI: 10.1212/WNL.0000000000001182

[21] Voinescu PE, Park S, Chen LQ, et al. Antiepileptic drug clearances during pregnancy and clinical implications for women with epilepsy. Neurology. 2018;**91**(13):e1228-e1236. DOI: 10.1212/WNL.0000000000006240

[22] Vlasov PN. Chapter 5. Epilepsy. In: Vlasov PN, Petrukhin VA, Avkhlediani KN, Lubnin AU, editors. Neurological Pathology and Pregnancy. Moscow: MEDPRESS-Inform; 2022. pp. 92-102. DOI: 10.24421/v4294-7741-1383-x

[23] Dmitrenko DV, Schnaider NA, Goroshkin AN, Tomilina AI, Vlasov PN, Sapronova MR. Russian register of pregnancy and epilepsy. Neurology, Neuropsychiatry, Psychosomatics. 2017;**9**(1c):21-25. DOI: 10.14412/2074-2711-2017-1S-21-25

[24] Pennell PB, Klein AM, Browning N, et al. Differential effects of antiepileptic drugs on neonatal outcomes. Epilepsy & Behavior. 2012;**24**(4):449-456. DOI: 10.1016/j.yebeh.2012.05.010

[25] Tomson T, Battino D, Bonizzoni E, et al. Comparative risk of major congenital malformations with eight different antiepileptic drugs: A prospective cohort study of the EURAP registry. Lancet Neurology. 2018;**17**(6):530-538. DOI: 10.1016/S1474-4422(18)30107-8

[26] Hernandez-Diaz S, Smith CR, Shen A, et al. Comparative safety of antiepileptic drugs during pregnancy. Neurology. 2012;**78**(21):1692-1699. DOI: 10.1212/WNL.0b013e3182574f39

[27] Campbell E, Kennedy F, Russell A, et al. Malformation risks of antiepileptic drug monotherapies in pregnancy: Updated results from the UK and Ireland Epilepsy and Pregnancy Registers. Journal of Neurology,

Neurosurgery, and Psychiatry. 2014;**85**(9):1029-1034

[28] Vajda FJ, O'Brien TJ, Lander CM, Graham J, Eadie MJ. The teratogenicity of the newer antiepileptic drugs—An update. Acta Neurologica Scandinavica. 2014;**130**:234-238. DOI: 10.1111/ane.12280

[29] Blotière PO, Raguideau F, Weill A, et al. Risks of 23 specific malformations associated with prenatal exposure to 10 antiepileptic drugs. Neurology. 2019;**93**(2):e167-e180. DOI: 10.1212/WNL.0000000000007696

[30] Veiby G, Daltveit AK, Schjolberg S, et al. Exposure to antiepileptic drugs in utero and child development: A prospective population-based study. Epilepsia. 2013;**54**(8):1462-1472. DOI: 10.1111/epi.12226

[31] Meador KJ, Baker GA, Browning N, et al. Foetal antiepileptic drug exposure and verbal versus non-verbal abilities at three years of age. Brain. 2011;**134**(2):396-404. DOI: 10.1093/brain/awq352

[32] Bromley RL, Calderbank R, Cheyne CP, et al. Cognition in school-age children exposed to levetiracetam, topiramate, or sodium valproate. Neurology. 2016;**87**(18):1943-1953. DOI: 10.1212/WNL.0000000000003157

[33] Huber-Mollema Y, Oort FJ, Lindhout D, Rodenburg R. Behavioral problems in children of mothers with epilepsy prenatally exposed to valproate, carbamazepine, lamotrigine, or levetiracetam monotherapy. Epilepsia. 2019;**60**(6):1069-1082

[34] Bromley RL, Weston J, Adab N, et al. Treatment for epilepsy in pregnancy: Neurodevelopmental outcomes in the child. Cochrane Database of Systematic Reviews. 2014;**10**:CD010236. DOI: 10.1002/14651858.CD010236.pub2

[35] Meador KJ, Baker GA, Browning N, et al. Breastfeeding in children of women taking antiepileptic drugs: Cognitive outcomes at age 6 years. JAMA Pediatrics. 2014;**168**(8):729-736. DOI: 10.1001/jamapediatrics.2014.118

[36] Elkjaer LS, Bech BH, Sun Y, Laursen TM, Christensen J. Association between prenatal valproate exposure and performance on standardized language and mathematics tests in school-aged children. JAMA Neurology. 2018;**75**(6):663-671. DOI: 10.1001/jamaneurol.2017.5035

[37] Bromley RL, Mawer GE, Briggs M, et al. The prevalence of neurodevelopmental disorders in children prenatally exposed to antiepileptic drugs. Journal of Neurology, Neurosurgery, and Psychiatry. 2013;**84**(6):637-643. DOI: 10.1136/jnnp-2012-304270

[38] Avakyan GN, Blinov DV, Avakyan GG, et al. Limitations of the use of valproic acid in girls and women: Expansion of contraindications in the instructions for medical use based on real clinical practice data. Epilepsy and Paroxysmal Conditions. 2019;**11**(2):110-123

[39] Czeizel AE, Dudas I, Vereczkey A, Banhidy F. Folate deficiency and folic acid supplementation: The prevention of neural-tube defects and congenital heart defects. Nutrients. 2013;**5**(11):4760-4775. DOI: 10.3390/nu5114760

[40] Bjork M, Riedel B, Spigset O, et al. Association of folic acid supplementation during pregnancy with the risk of autistic traits in children exposed to antiepileptic drugs in utero. JAMA Neurology.

2018;**75**(2):160-168. DOI: 10.1001/jamaneurol.2017.3897

[41] Husebye ES, Gilhus NE, Riedel B, Spigset O, Daltveit AK, Bjork MH. Verbal abilities in children of mothers with epilepsy: Association to maternal folate status. Neurology. 2018;**91**(9):e811-e821. DOI: 10.1212/WNL.0000000000006073

[42] Harden CL, Pennell PB, Koppel BS, et al. Management issues for women with epilepsy--focus on pregnancy (an evidence-based review): III. Vitamin K, folic acid, blood levels, and breast-feeding: Report of the quality standards subcommittee and therapeutics and technology assessment Subcommittee of the American Academy of neurology and the American Epilepsy Society. Epilepsia. 2009;**50**(5):1247-1255. DOI: 10.1111/j.1528-1167.2009.02130.x

[43] Murray LK, Smith MJ, Jadavji NM. Maternal oversupplementation with folic acid and its impact on neurodevelopment of offspring. Nutrition Reviews. 2018;**76**(9):708-721. DOI: 10.1093/nutrit/nuy025

[44] Reimers A, Helde G, Bråthen G, Brodtkorb E. Lamotrigine and its N2-glucuronide during pregnancy: The significance of renal clearance and estradiol. Epilepsy Research. 2011;**94**(3):198-205. DOI: 10.1016/j.eplepsyres.2011.02.002

[45] Karanam A, Pennell PB, French JA, et al. Lamotrigine clearance increases by 5 weeks gestational age: Relationship to estradiol concentrations and gestational age. Annals of Neurology. 2018;**84**(4):556-563. DOI: 10.1002/ana.25321

[46] Minicucci F, Ferlisi M, Brigo F, Mecarelli O, Meletti S, Aguglia U, et al. Management of status epilepticus in adults. Position paper of the Italian league against epilepsy. Epilepsy & Behavior. 2020:102. DOI: 10.1016/j.yebeh.2019.106675

[47] Vlasov PN, Drojina GR, Petrukchin VA, Grishin VL, Melnikov AP. Haemostatic parameters of newborns from mothers with epilepsy. Epileptologia. 2012;**20**(1):5-9

[48] Tomson T, Battino D, Bromley R, et al. Global survey of guidelines for the Management of Epilepsy in pregnancy: A report from the international league against epilepsy task force on women and pregnancy. Epilepsia Open. 2020;**5**:366-370. DOI: 10.1002/epi4.12420

Section 2

Epileptic Syndromes

Chapter 4

Perspective Chapter: Red Flags for Syndromic Epilepsy

Bita Shalbafan

Abstract

Despite the high frequency of seizures and propensity to develop status epilepticus (SE) most cases do not develop a long-term predisposition to seizures. So, investigating a patient with refractory epilepsy or unexplained status epilepticus is important to consider the possibility of treatable diseases i.e. treatable types of inborn error of metabolism, paraneoplasia, infections, and TLE due to temporal lobe encephalocele and IIH. Epilepsy syndrome (ES) refers to a cluster of features that should be paying attention to its red flags to narrow the wide differential diagnosis.

Keywords: syndromic epilepsy, paraneoplasia, inborn error of metabolism, encephaloceles, new-onset refractory status epilepticus

1. Introduction

Epilepsy can be observed during the course of many usually as part of a large clinical spectrum. Epilepsy Syndrome diagnosis step-by-step approach starts in the first level to detect seizure type semiologically, then Epilepsy type detection as the second level, *epilepsy syndrome* (ES) is diagnosed based on any co-morbidity in the third level [1].

1.1 Definition

An epilepsy syndrome (ES) refers to a group of features that includes seizure types, EEG, and imaging features that tend to occur together. There are many well-known syndromes, such as childhood absence epilepsy, West syndrome, and Dravet syndrome, although it should be noted that there has never been a formal classification of syndromes. Therefore, it is important to note that epilepsy syndrome does not have a one-to-one correlation with an etiological diagnosis and serves a different purpose, such as guiding management [1].

2. Epilepsy syndrome diagnosis

2.1 When should one suspect an epileptic syndrome?

On analyzing the history, the following keys are to be identified for a syndromic diagnosis [1]:

Mixture of generalized and partial epilepsy; special seizure types i.e. temporal lobe epilepsy or myoclonic epilepsy; association with other impairments i.e. neurological impairments, mental retardation, other organ disorders (eyes, muscles spleen, etc.); seizures related to the times of eating, fasting, protein-rich meal; unexplained Status epilepticus; inefficacy or worsening with classical antiepileptic drugs; and paraclinical Findings.

2.1.1 Diagnostic approach to syndromic epilepsy

2.1.1.1 Disease course

One of the most important points that should be noted in the history of an epileptic patient is the *disease course*. Non-progressive course suggests a static nature of disorders like stroke, chromosomal diseases, perinatal hypoxia, etc. On the other hand, starting and tempered profiles in progressive disorders play three patterns:

Acute: The presence of abrupt and severe symptoms, along with periods of improvement and worsening, a connection to infections, fasting, or specific dietary habits, non-specific physical indications, and a positive reaction to symptomatic treatment, frequently indicates a deficiency in intermediary metabolisms, such as aminoacidopathies, organic acidemias, and fatty acid oxidation disorders.

Insidious onset: A gradual onset, persistent and progressive symptoms, and symptoms and signs that are independent of intervening events often suggest organelle disorders such as lysosomal storage disorders and peroxisomal disorders.

Episodic progression of symptoms: There are exceptions to this generalization. For example, Leigh's disease, which is an organelle disease, is characterized by a sudden onset of encephalopathy and an episodic course [2].

2.1.1.2 Extra-neural involvements

1. If a person has unusual physical characteristics in their fingers, face, spine, toes, extremities, or internal organs, it may indicate that these features developed before birth. Coarse facial features are often associated with mucopolysaccharidoses, GM1 gangliosidoses, mucolipidoses, and glycoprotein syndromes such as fucosidosis. Children with hyperhomocystinuria may have a Marfanoid habitus [2].

2. Skin and hair abnormalities can provide valuable information for diagnosing systemic diseases that affect the nervous system. For example:

    - A child with sparse, light-colored hair, hair loss, and recurring skin rashes, along with regression and seizures that do not respond to treatment, may have biotinidase deficiency;

    - A child with seborrheic dermatitis, hypopigmented kinky hair, epilepsy, and regression in early infancy is immediately diagnosed with Menkes disease;

    - *hypertrichosis* is a feature of mitochondrial disorders, especially in *SURF1*-positive Leigh disease.

    - A child has spastic paraplegia and leukoencephalopathy on an MRI, along with ichthyosis (a scaly skin condition), which may indicate Sjogren Larsson syndrome.

- Angiokeratomas, which are small, dark red or purple spots on the skin, can be observed in both Fabry's disease and fucosidosis.
- Cutaneous melanosis, which is an abnormal darkening of the skin, is another important clinical clue in patients with lysosomal storage disorders, particularly GM1 gangliosidosis.
- hyperpigmentation of the oral mucosa, genitals, and navel in a child with regression of milestones may indicate a diagnosis of adrenoleukodystrophy [2, 3].

3. Measurement of head circumference and velocity of growth is an important aspect of a clinical examination and can provide valuable diagnostic information. For example:
    - If a child has an abnormally large head (macrocephaly) and exhibits a startling response to sound, along with regression at around six months of age, may indicate a diagnosis of GM2 gangliosidosis.
    - Extreme irritability, incessant crying, opisthotonic posture, and regression are diagnostic clues to Krabbe disease.
    - In glutaric aciduria type 1, episodic regression occurs after febrile illnesses, especially mild diarrheal illnesses, together with macrocephaly and dystonia.
    - In a child with suspected leukodystrophy, a large head suggests a variety of diagnoses such as Canavans disease, Alexander disease, and megalencephalic leukodystrophy with subcortical cysts.
    - Macrocephaly can also be seen in another important late-onset metabolic disorder, L-2-hydroxyglutaric aciduria, in which there is evidence of leukoencephalopathy on MRI [2–4].

4. The eye is often referred to as a "window to the brain". This is because the eye is connected to the brain through the optic nerve, which carries visual information from the eye to the brain. By examining the eye, doctors can sometimes detect changes or abnormalities in the brain that may be indicative of certain medical conditions [2, 5].
    - *Ocular anterior chamber examination:* The main points to look for are the presence of cataracts, lens luxation, and corneal opacity. When children present with progressive extrapyramidal signs, it is important to look for the Kayser Fleisher ring to establish a diagnosis of Wilson's disease. The presence of lens dislocation in a child with refractory neonatal-onset epilepsy may indicate isolated sulfite oxidase deficiency or molybdenum co-factor deficiency. In contrast, lens dislocation in a child with mental retardation, behavioral disturbances, and Marfanoid habitus may suggest homocystinuria. Corneal opacity is a characteristic feature of cerebrotendinous xanthomatosis, mucopolysaccharidoses, and mucolipidosis type 4. In these disorders, corneal opacity may be associated with ptosis, oculomotor disorders, retinal degeneration, optic atrophy, and spastic atactic syndrome. MRI may reveal a thin corpus callosum

and variable degrees of hypomyelination. However, visceromegaly and skeletal manifestations are typically absent in these children.

- *Ocular posterior chamber examination:* Changes in the appearance of the optic nerve can be a sign of increased pressure in the brain, which may be caused by conditions such as a brain tumor or hydrocephalus. Retinitis pigmentosa, optic atrophy, papilledema, and cherry red spots. Pigment disorders of the retina often occur in diseases of the mitochondria, neuronal ceroid lipofuscinoses, and disorders of peroxisomal biogenesis. Cherry-red spots typically appear in lysosomal storage disorders such as Tay-Sachs disease, Niemann-Pick type C disease, and GM1 gangliosidosis. As a novel and non-invasive tool, Optic Coherence Tomography findings will evaluate papilledema in epileptic cases.

- *Ocular eye movement examination:* Certain eye movements and reflexes can provide clues about the functioning of the brainstem, which is responsible for controlling many vital functions such as breathing and heart rate. *Vertical supranuclear gaze palsy* may suggest Niemann Pick type C disease.

3. Etiologies of syndromic epilepsy

3.1 Structural

It is important for neurologists, particularly epileptologists, and those working on multidisciplinary epilepsy teams to recognize the link between structural brain abnormalities and epilepsy. Tumors, trauma, bleeding, abscesses, and encephalitis can be difficult to detect with conventional imaging methods [6]. In some cases, imaging with 3 T MRI and high-resolution CT of the skull base may be required to confirm temporal lobe sclerosis and encephaloceles, particularly in patients with nonlesional temporal lobe epilepsy (TLE). Treatment of drug-resistant TLE due to temporal lobe encephalocele and sclerosis is primarily surgical and most patients have a good outcome (postoperative Engel Class I).

Temporal lobe encephaloceles are increasingly recognized as a cause of epilepsy. Recent studies have found an association between temporal lobe encephalocele and IIH, suggesting that TLE may be an unusual manifestation or complication of IIH. It has been suggested that pulsatile forces in the cerebrospinal fluid (CSF) due to increased intracranial pressure can lead to the development of prominent arachnoid villi that form CSF pockets, leading to the formation of spontaneous CSF fistulas and encephaloceles [7].

Patients with temporal lobe epilepsy (TLE) and temporal lobe encephalocele have similar demographic characteristics as patients with idiopathic intracranial hypertension (IIH); including female dominance and high body mass index (BMI). Several studies have also shown a high prevalence of raised intracranial pressure (RAD-IH) in patients with TLE and temporal lobe encephalocele, including enlarged or empty sella, enlarged Meckel's cavity, optic nerve sheath distension, flattening of the posterior bulb, and transverse venous sinus stenosis. Other symptoms and signs of IIH, such as headache, visual disturbances, pulsatile tinnitus, and papilledema, are rare in patients with TLE and temporal lobe encephalocele. However, some patients with TLE and temporal lobe encephalocele have elevated cerebrospinal fluid (CSF) opening pressure greater than 25 cm H_2O, supporting an association with IIH [7–14].

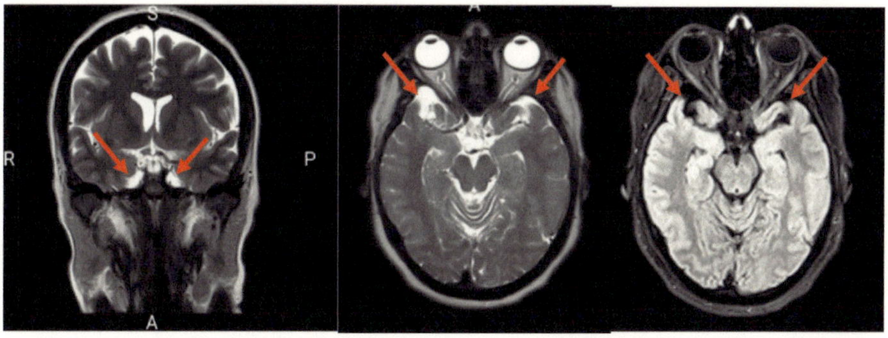

Figure 1.
Bilateral encephaloceles showing by red arrows in brain MRI (a) T2 weighted coronal cut; (b) T2 weighted axial cut at the same level; (c) T1 weighted axial cut at the same level (Bita Shalbafan courtesy).

In a large series of 474 patients examined over 5 years in a center for epilepsy surgery, temporal lobe encephalocele was identified in 25 (5.3%) patients. In these patients, the temporal lobe encephalocele was regarded as an epileptogenic focus in 48% of the cases. Temporal lobe encephaloceles are thought to cause mechanical irritation of the temporal lobes, and secondary changes such as inflammation and gliosis serve as a starting point for seizures. Most temporal lobe encephaloceles are asymptomatic and are discovered incidentally in patients with no history of seizures. However, in a small proportion of patients with drug-resistant temporal lobe epilepsy, temporal lobe encephaloceles associated with an anterior middle fossa defect (anteromedial and anteroinferior temporal lobe encephaloceles) appear to lateralize to the side of seizure onset, showing high concordance with studies including PET, scalp EEG and seizure semiology (**Figure 1**) [7–14].

3.2 Infectious diseases

Various infections of the central nervous system can cause both acute seizures and epilepsy. The pathogenesis and clinical presentation of seizure disorders can vary significantly depending on the infectious agent. The exact mechanisms underlying these differences are not well understood, but they appear to be at least partially related to factors such as the type of pathogen, the extent of cortical involvement, delays in treatment, and the host's inflammatory response.

Acute viral encephalitis can be caused by a variety of viruses, including herpes viruses, enteroviruses, paramyxoviruses, and arthropod-borne and zoonotic viruses. Some of the most common viruses associated with acute viral encephalitis include [15, 16]:

Herpes simplex virus type 1: This is the most commonly diagnosed sporadic encephalitis.

Enterovirus 71: This virus is associated with epidemic hand, foot, and mouth disease, aseptic meningitis, brainstem encephalitis, and myelitis.

Measles virus: This virus can cause acute post-infective encephalitis, subacute encephalitis, and subacute sclerosing panencephalitis.

West Nile virus: This virus is found in North America, Southern Europe, the Middle East, and West and Central Asia, and is associated with flaccid paralysis and Parkinsonian movement disorders.

Disease	Parasite	Transmitted by
Neurocysticercosis	*Taenia solium*	pork
Malaria	*Plasmodium falciparum*	mosquitoes
Toxoplasmosis	*Toxoplasma gondii*	cat
Schistosomiasis	*Schistosoma*	freshwater snail
Trypanosomiasis	*Trypanosoma*	tsetse fly

Table 1.
Seizure-induced parasitic infections.

Japanese encephalitis virus: This virus is found in Asia and is associated with flaccid paralysis and Parkinsonian movement disorders.

Rabies virus: This virus is transmitted by dogs, cats, and bats, depending on the location.

Other viruses that can cause acute viral encephalitis include varicella-zoster virus, Epstein-Barr virus, cytomegalovirus, mumps virus, and tick-borne encephalitis virus. It is important to note that viral causes of chronic encephalitis, such as JC virus, are not included in this list. A thorough evaluation by a neurologist or other specialist is necessary to determine the underlying cause of encephalitis and develop an appropriate management plan.

It is important to note that while these parasitic infections can cause seizures, they are relatively rare in developed countries (**Table 1**) [15, 16].

3.3 Autoimmune diseases and paraneoplasia

Despite the high seizure frequency and propensity to develop status epilepticus (SE) in the acute stage of autoimmune encephalitis (AE), most patients with AE do not develop a long-term predisposition to seizures. This important concept was highlighted by the International League Against Epilepsy (ILAE) in 2020 when the Autoimmunity and Inflammation Taskforce proposed two main diagnostic entities: "acute symptomatic seizures secondary to AE" and "autoimmune-associated epilepsy". The latter occurs in a minority of cases and is often due to the development of structural abnormalities after the resolution of the inflammation (eg, mesial temporal sclerosis) or to a persistent antigenic trigger (eg, cancer in paraneoplastic cases). The amount of new information in this area over the last decade regarding clinical specifics, laboratory diagnostics, and treatment options has made it difficult for neurologists to target patients with AEs and seizures [17–21].

The predisposition to cause enduring seizures in autoimmune encephalitis is dependent on the mechanism that drives the immune response, ranging from a high predisposition in cytotoxic T cell-mediated encephalitis (intracellular antigens) to a moderate or absent predisposition in antibody-mediated encephalitis (surface antigens). Among the latter, the severity of the seizures and the likelihood of developing epilepsy vary according to the antigen. Additionally, all these disorders occur with a variable degree of inflammation that could have downstream effects on synaptic function, hyperexcitability, and epileptogenesis. Several autoimmune antibodies to: Glutamate/NMDA-NR1, Glutamate/AMPA-GluR3, Glutamate/NMDA-NR2, GABA-R, GAD-65, GLY-R, LGI1, VGKC, CASPR2, and β2 GP1, found in subpopulations of epilepsy patients. AMPA-GluR3B peptide antibodies as Glutamate receptor antibodies seem so far the most

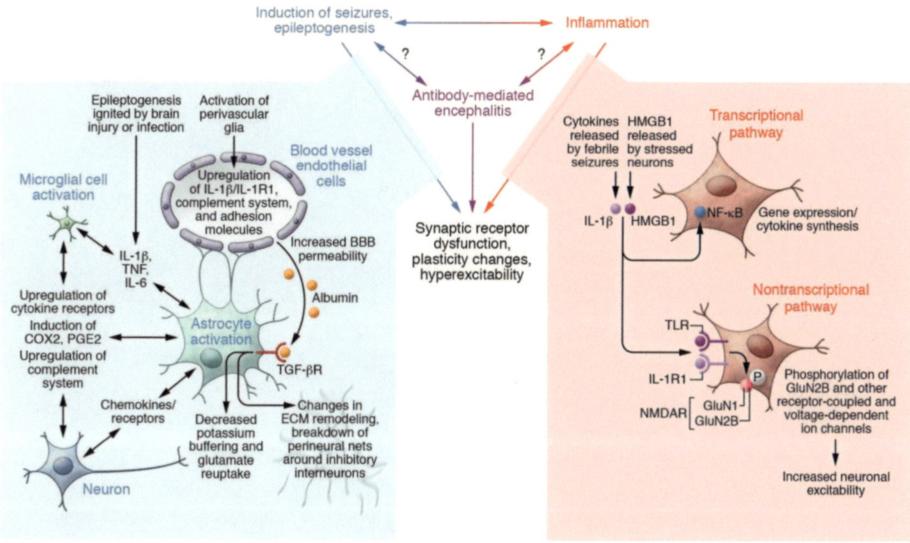

Figure 2.
Multiple inflammatory/innate immunity mechanisms triggered by seizures and epileptogenesis.

exclusive and pathogenic autoimmune antibodies in AE. They kill neural cells by three mechanisms: reactive-oxygen-species, excitotoxicity, and complement fixation, and facilitate and/or induce brain damage, seizures, and behavioral impairments. Also, the additional autoantibodies GABA-R, dopamine-R, Ach-R, adrenergic-R, and serotonin-R are present in various neurological diseases (**Figure 2**) [17–21].

From a clinical perspective, only a few seizure types are pathognomonic for an autoimmune etiology, including faciobrachial dystonic seizures (FBDS) and seizures originating in perisylvian (islet-opercular) regions. FBDS are very brief (<3 s) tonic muscle contractions in the arm and face, and more rarely in the leg. They are usually unilateral, but can also independently affect both sides asynchronously and occur up to 100 times a day, including during sleep. FBDS are thought to be pathognomonic of anti-LGI1 encephalitis, and their early detection (and consequent initiation of immunotherapy, particularly corticosteroids) can prevent the onset of cognitive dysfunction characteristic of the disease. Seizures with perisylvian semiology, including autonomic and somatosensory/viscerosensory symptoms, are not associated with a specific antibody but are often indicative of an immune-mediated etiology. A multicenter study found that autoimmune etiologies were more common than infection in NORSE (new-onset refractory status epilepticus), with autoimmune etiologies comprising 19% nonparaneoplastic and 18% paraneoplastic cases. These results suggest that autoimmune pathogenesis is much more likely in NORSE than viral infection. Therefore, after a thorough investigation of the infection, it is possible to consider NORSE as a potentially autoimmune epilepsy that requires active immunotherapy. A similar condition has been described in children, which is defined as febrile infectious epilepsy syndrome (FIRES). In these cases, the presence of a febrile episode between 2 weeks and 24 hours before the onset of RSE is required. Some authors argue that NORSE and FIRES are different entities. However, the two syndromes share many similarities and nowadays FIRES is considered a subcategory of NORSE (**Figure 3**) [17–21].

Timely identification of an autoimmune cause of seizures is crucial as it has relevant therapeutic implications. Several criteria and scoring systems for autoimmune

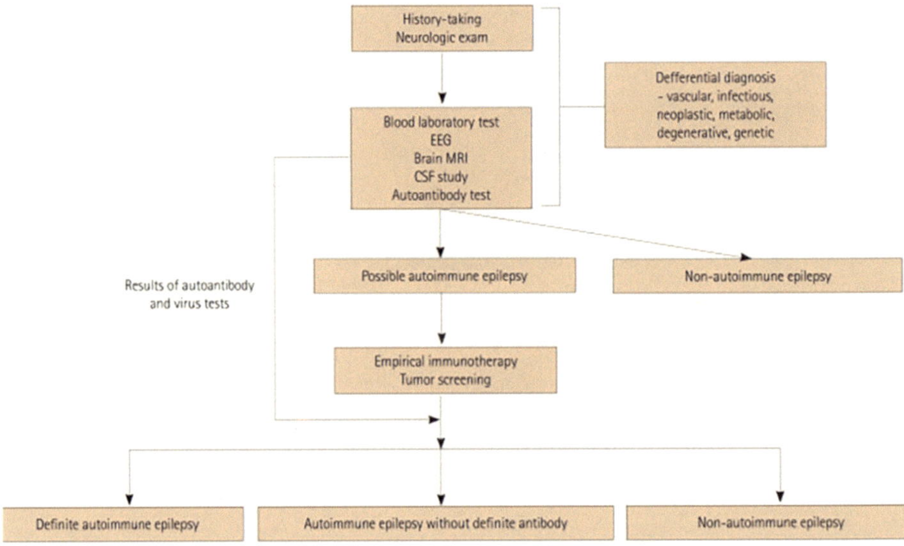

Figure 3.
The diagnostic approach to autoimmune epilepsy begins with a detailed history-taking and neurological examination. To exclude other etiologies of epilepsy, various diagnostic workups including blood laboratory tests, electroencephalography (EEG), brain magnetic resonance imaging (MRI), and cerebrospinal fluid (CSF) studies are performed. Empirical immunotherapy can be applied during the diagnostic tests. The final diagnosis is made based on the results of the tests and the response to immunotherapy. Blood laboratory tests may include autoimmune antibody panels, complete blood count, erythrocyte sedimentation rate, C-reactive protein, and liver and kidney function tests. EEG can help identify seizure activity and epileptiform discharges. Brain MRI can detect structural abnormalities and inflammation. CSF studies can detect inflammation and the presence of specific antibodies. Empirical immunotherapy may include corticosteroids, intravenous immunoglobulin, or plasma exchange. The response to immunotherapy can help confirm the diagnosis of autoimmune epilepsy.

seizures and epilepsy have been proposed, such as the Autoantibody Prevalence in Epilepsy Score (APE) and its subsequent revision (APE2), the Antibody Contribution to Focal Epilepsy Signs and Symptoms (ACES) score, and others. A clinician should be certain that the panel chosen includes antibodies for the suspected etiology (**Table 2**) and screen for antibodies associated with conditions that present similarly (ie, GQ1B, ANA, and TPO/thyroglobulin antibodies) [17, 18].

3.4 Inborn errors of metabolism (IEMs)

Although IEMs are a rare etiology in child and adult epileptic cases, these are important to recognize for several reasons: dramatic response to specific treatments; early treatment can stop disease progression in neural and extra-neural tissues; some antiepileptic drugs interfering with metabolic pathways may worsen the clinical condition; specific genetic counseling can be provided.

When a metabolic disease is suspected, the approach to metabolic investigations should be guided by the type of epilepsy, associated signs, and the presence or absence of mental retardation. In critical situations, such as an unexplained status epilepticus, ammonia measurement and search for porphyries should be mandatory. In other situations, simple examinations aimed at identifying treatable diseases should be seen as a priority. Metabolic investigations may include blood tests to assess electrolyte levels, glucose, liver and kidney function, and thyroid

Autonomic dysfunction: atrial bradycardia or sustained tachycardia, blood pressure labile, bradycardia, cardiac aystole, hyperhidrosis, orthostatic hypotension, ventricular tachycardia.	1
Brain MRI: consistent with limbic encephalitis (medial temporal T2/FLAIR signal changes)	2
Seizure or cognitive changes: rapidly progressive mental changes over 1–6 week period or new onset seizure (within 1 year of evaluation)	1
CSF findings consistent with inflammation: protein >50 mg/dL and lymphocytic pleocytosis >5 cells/dL, if total number of red blood cells is <1000 cells/dL	2
Facial dyskinesia or faciobrachial dystonia	2
Malignancy (excludes cutaneous basal cell carcinoma or squamous cell carcinoma)	2
Psychiatric symptoms (agitation, aggression, emotional lability)	1
Seizure refractory to medical treatment	2
Viral prodrome (low-grade fever, sore throat, rhinorrhea); scored only if there is no underlying malignancy	2

Note. An APE Score of ≥4 (max: 15) predicts detection of neural autoantibody in autoimmune epilepsy (sensitivity: 97.7%,; specificity: 77.9%) [17].
Abbreviations: CSF, cerebrospinal fluid; FLAIR, fluid-attenuated inversion recovery.

Table 2.
Autoantibody prevalence in epilepsy score.

function. Urine tests may also be performed to assess for metabolic abnormalities. Genetic testing may be considered in patients with suspected inherited metabolic disorders. In patients with suspected mitochondrial disorders, muscle biopsy may be necessary to assess mitochondrial function. Magnetic resonance spectroscopy (MRS) can also be used to evaluate brain metabolism and detect metabolic abnormalities. It is important to note that metabolic investigations should be conducted in consultation with a metabolic specialist or neurologist with expertise in metabolic disorders, as the interpretation of results can be complex and require specialized knowledge (**Figure 4**) [2, 19].

To recognize the type of IEM clinical history needs to be analyzed considering the following points [2]:

3.4.1 Pattern of inheritance

- *Autosomal dominant traits* can be present in successive generations, although the level of expressivity can vary.

- *Autosomal recessive traits* are often not manifested in consecutive generations but may be present in siblings. Almost 90% of metabolic disorders are inherited in an autosomal recessive manner. Because of the little siblings, cases appear to be sporadic at times. A family history of unexplained neonatal or infant deaths should be obtained.

- *X-linked recessive* disorders manifest in male siblings, male first cousins, and maternal uncles, e.g. B. Fabry disease, X-linked adrenoleukodystrophy, and Lesch-Nyhan disease.

A maternal inheritance pattern suggests a mitochondrial disorder, which is caused by mutations in the mitochondrial DNA (mtDNA) that is inherited from the mother. It is important to note that mitochondrial disorders can also follow a Mendelian

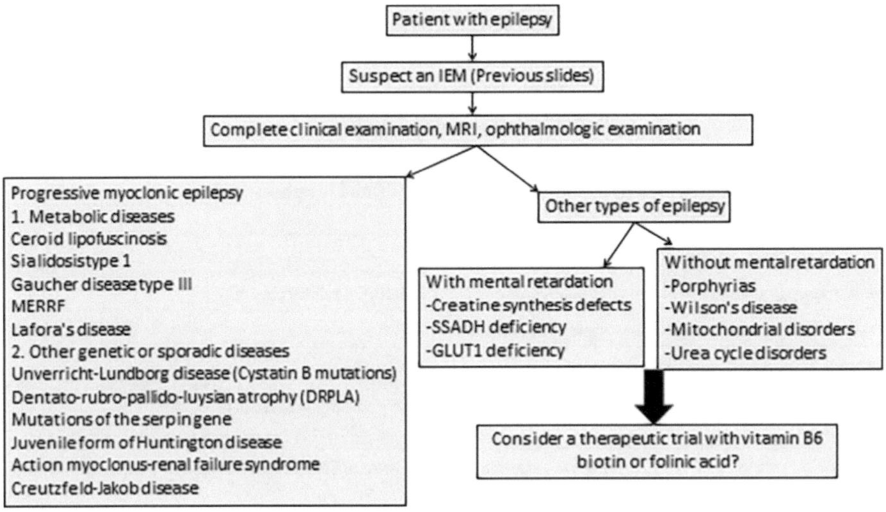

Figure 4.
Diagnostic approach in an epileptic patient in order not to miss an IEM summarize presumed hereditary predisposition critical problem of inherited stigma in some parts of the world causes us to prefer the idiopathic labeling to these epileptic cases instead of genetic names. Also, findings of many de novo mutations cannot confirm the pathogenicity of these genetic findings in both mild and severe epilepsies.

pattern of inheritance, such as autosomal dominant or recessive inheritance, depending on the specific mutation and the proportion of mutant mtDNA in the affected individual.

In some cases, an apparent autosomal inheritance pattern may mask a maternal inheritance. This can occur when a mutation in the mtDNA is present in both the mother and father, but the father's contribution of mtDNA to the offspring is much lower than the mother's. As a result, the offspring may appear to inherit the mutation in an autosomal dominant or recessive pattern, when in fact it is a mitochondrial disorder with maternal inheritance.

Therefore, when evaluating a patient with suspected mitochondrial disorder, it is important to consider both the maternal inheritance pattern and the possibility of Mendelian inheritance. Genetic testing, including mtDNA sequencing and analysis of nuclear genes involved in mitochondrial function, may be necessary to confirm the diagnosis and determine the mode of inheritance (**Table 3**) [2].

It is important to recognize that the clinical presentation and imaging features of the same disease can vary in different age groups. Therefore, it is essential to be familiar with the variable presentation of these disorders in different age groups to make an accurate diagnosis and develop an appropriate management plan. For example, Tay Sachs disease or infantile GM2 gangliosidosis typically presents with neuroregression and an exaggerated startle response to sounds. In contrast, the presentation of juvenile-onset GM2 gangliosidosis includes neuroregression, gait difficulty, ataxia, peripheral neuropathy, and psychosis. The classical early infantile Krabbe leukodystrophy presents with regression, irritable cry, and opisthotonic posturing, while juvenile onset Krabbe leukodystrophy presents with spastic paraparesis or visual impairment. In addition to the clinical presentation, the magnetic resonance imaging (MRI) findings can also vary in different age groups. For example, in early infantile Krabbe leukodystrophy, MRI typically shows diffuse white matter abnormalities, while in juvenile-onset Krabbe leukodystrophy, MRI may show focal white matter

Diagnosis	Onset	Seizure type	Nonepileptic clinical findings	Diagnostic evaluation
Glycine encephalopathy	Neonatal period to early infancy	Myoclonic jerks, infantile spasm	—	Elevated glycine on TMS and quantitative estimation of amino acids
Isolated sulfite oxidase/ Molybdenum cofactor deficiency	Neonatal period to early infancy	Refractory seizure	Presentation similar to hypoxic ischemia encephalopathy, facial dysmorphism, lens dislocation	Low serum uric acid, positive urine sulfite testing
Maple syrup urine disease	Neonatal period to early infancy	GTS	Encephalopathy, abnormal smell of the body and urine	Elevated branched-chain amino acids on TMS, urinary DNPH test-positive
Phenylketonuria	Early infancy to childhood	Infantile spasms,	Hypopigmented hair, abnormal smell of urine, microcephaly	Elevated phenylalanine on TMS/HPLC, positive ferric chloride, and DNPH test
Menkes kinky hair syndrome	Early infancy to childhood	Focal clonic seizures, infantile spasms, myoclonic seizures	Hypopigmented kinky and friable hair, hypotonia, seborrheic dermatitis	Low serum copper and ceruloplasmin levels, hair microscopy-pili Torti
Biotinidase deficiency	Early infancy	Infantile spasms, refractory myoclonic seizures	Alopecia, hypopigmentation of hair	Elevated C5-OH levels on TMS, elevated beta hydroxyl isovalerate, methyl citrate, and beta hydroxy propionate and lactate on urinary organic acid analysis, dramatic response to biotin
Progressive neuronal degeneration [Alpers disease/ polymerase gamma (POLG) related disorder]	Late infancy to early childhood	GTC, myoclonic jerks	Transient hemiplegia, fatal hepatic encephalopathy especially after sodium valproate use	Elevated liver enzymes, POLG1 genetic study,

Table 3.
Neurometabolic disorders with epilepsy as the main manifestation.

abnormalities. Therefore, a thorough evaluation by a neurologist or other specialist is necessary to make an accurate diagnosis and develop an appropriate management plan, taking into account the age of the patient and the variable presentation of the disorder in different age groups [2].

3.4.2 Key clinical symptoms and signs with special focus on sites of neuraxis

When evaluating a patient with a suspected neurological disorder, it is important to determine whether the primary symptoms and signs are related to gray matter involvement, white matter involvement, behavioral or psychiatric manifestations, extrapyramidal system involvement, or peripheral nerve system involvement. Gray matter involvement can present with symptoms such as seizures, visual impairment, and cognitive decline. Examples of disorders that primarily involve gray matter include epilepsy, Alzheimer's disease, and Huntington's disease. White matter involvement can present with symptoms such as gait difficulty, abnormalities in tone (spasticity/hypotonia), and sensory deficits. Examples of disorders that primarily involve white matter include leukodystrophies, multiple sclerosis, and cerebral palsy. Behavioral or psychiatric manifestations can present with symptoms such as aggression, irritability, and anxiety. Examples of disorders that primarily involve behavioral or psychiatric manifestations include autism spectrum disorder, attention-deficit/hyperactivity disorder (ADHD), and schizophrenia. Extrapyramidal system involvement can present with symptoms such as dystonia, tremor, and choreoathetosis. Examples of disorders that primarily involve the extrapyramidal system include Parkinson's disease, Huntington's disease, and dystonia. Peripheral nerve system involvement can present with symptoms such as polyneuropathy and pes cavus. Examples of disorders that primarily involve the peripheral nerve system include Charcot-Marie-Tooth disease and hereditary neuropathies. Therefore, a thorough evaluation by a neurologist or other specialist is necessary to determine the primary symptoms and signs and develop an appropriate management plan based on the underlying pathology [2].

3.4.2.1 Association with extraneural impairments

It was explained in detail in part 2.1.1.2.

3.4.2.2 Progressive myoclonic epilepsy

This is a group of disorders characterized by a specific set of clinical features, electroencephalography (EEG) findings, and response to treatment. However, in some cases, the clinical presentation of epilepsy may not match with any classical ES. This is known as an atypical electro-clinical presentation. Atypical electro-clinical presentation can refer to a variety of features, including an unusual combination of seizure types, an unusual age of onset, or an unusual response to antiepileptic drugs. For example, a patient may present with a mixture of generalized and partial epileptic manifestations, such as the association of myoclonus and partial seizures in a given patient. In such cases, a thorough evaluation by a neurologist or other specialist is necessary to determine the underlying pathology and develop an appropriate management plan. This may include further diagnostic tests, such as brain imaging or genetic testing, to identify the cause of the atypical presentation. Treatment may involve a combination of antiepileptic drugs and other therapies, such as surgery or behavioral interventions, depending on the specific features of the atypical presentation. It is important to note that atypical electro-clinical presentation is relatively rare and may require specialized expertise to diagnose and manage. Therefore, referral to a specialist center or epilepsy center may be necessary in some cases (**Table 4**) [2].

3.4.2.3 Other red flags

Anti-epileptic drugs may exacerbate epilepsy or trigger a metabolic attack in patients with IEMs (**Table 5**) [20].

Diagnosis	Onset	Clinical features except seizure	MRI findings	Diagnostic evaluation
Neuronal ceroid lipofuscinosis	Infantile, late Infantile, juvenile adult onset	Rapidly advancing psychomotor retardation, ataxia, blindness, Retinitis Pigmentosa, optic atrophy	cerebral and cerebellar atrophy with periventricular signal changes	Giant somatosensory evoked potential, electron microscopy of axillary skin shows characteristic inclusion
Cherry red spot myoclonic syndrome	Late childhood to adolescence	GTCS, ataxia, cherry red spot	Nonspecific findings	Giant somatosensory evoked potential, Bone marrow storage cells
Myoclonic epilepsy ragged red fiber (MERRF) syndrome	Late childhood to adolescence and adulthood	Ataxia, intention tremor, Muscular weakness, deafness, optic atrophy	Nonspecific findings	Elevated lactate,Ragged red and blue fibers in muscle biopsy
Nieman Pick type C disease	Late childhood	Ataxia, cataplexy, supranuclear vertical gaze palsy, splenomegaly	Cerebellar atrophy	Bone marrow examination for storage cells,genetic testing
Gaucher disease type III	7–10 Y/O	psychomotor retardation, splenomegaly, osseous signs	Nonspecific findings	Glucocerebrosidase enzyme activity estimation by gottery test, bone marrow examination for storage cells
Late-onset GM2 gangliosidosis	4-10Y/O	Ataxia cherry red spots	Nonspecific findings	serum hexoseaminidase levels

TMS, Tendom Mass Spectroscopy; HPLC, High Performance Liquid Chromatography; MRS, Magnetic Resonance Spectroscopy.

Table 4.
Progressive myoclonic epilepsy syndromes.

Disease	Drugs that may exacerbate epilepsy or trigger a metabolic attack
Progressive myoclonic epilepsy (not specific to IEMs)	phenytoin, carbamazepine, gabapentin, vigabatrin, Tiagabine, lamotrigine
GLUT-1 deficiency	Diazepam, phenobarbital
SSADH deficiency	Valproate
Porphyrias	Valproate, lamotrigine, carbamazepine, phenytoin, topiramate
Urea cycle disorders	Valproate
Mitochondrial cytopathies	Valproate

Table 5.
List of IEMs that may be exacerbated by anti-epileptic drugs.

3.4.3 Paraclinic

Pattern of white matter abnormalities on magnetic resonance imaging (MRI) is one of the most important tools in the diagnosis of specific IEM types (**Figure 5**) [3]:

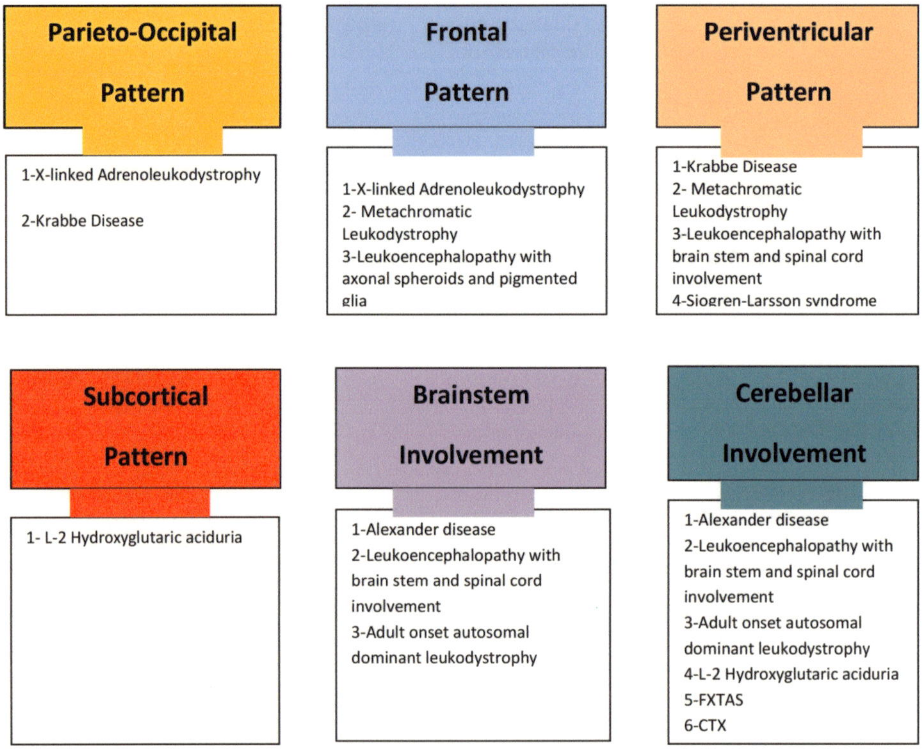

Figure 5.
Patterns of white matter abnormalities on magnetic resonance imaging (MRI) in IEM.

Abnormalities on *proton magnetic resonance spectroscopy*: for instance, creatine deficiency or increased in lactate in Mitochondrial disorders.

Electroencephalogram showing slowing of the background activity or photo-paroxysmal responses during the photic intermittent stimulation at low frequencies (1–6 H).

3.4.4 Treatable IEMs

When investigating a patient with refractory epilepsy or unexplained status epilepticus, it is important to consider the possibility of treatable diseases [20].

The following investigations may be considered:

1. Glucocerebrosidase activity: This test can help diagnose Gaucher disease, a rare genetic disorder that can cause seizures and other neurological symptoms.

2. Blood copper and ceruloplasmin: These tests can help diagnose Wilson's disease, a rare genetic disorder that can cause seizures and other neurological symptoms.

3. Blood and urine creatine (or proton magnetic resonance spectroscopy): These tests can help diagnose creatine deficiency syndromes, a group of rare genetic disorders that can cause seizures and other neurological symptoms.

4. Blood and CSF glucose (with calculation of the blood/CSF ratio): These tests can help diagnose hypoglycorrhachia, a condition in which the glucose level in the CSF is lower than expected. This can be caused by a variety of conditions, including infections, tumors, and metabolic disorders.

5. CSF lactate and search for mitochondrial disorders: These tests can help diagnose mitochondrial disorders, a group of rare genetic disorders that can cause seizures and other neurological symptoms.

6. In cases of refractory epilepsy or unexplained status epilepticus, a simple therapeutic trial with vitamin B6 (250 mg/day), biotin (10–300 mg/day), and folinic acid (25–50 mg/day) for several days or weeks may be considered. These vitamins can help improve seizure control in some patients with certain genetic disorders, such as pyridoxine-dependent epilepsy or biotinidase deficiency. It is important to note that these investigations should be conducted in consultation with a neurologist or other specialist with expertise in metabolic disorders, as the interpretation of results can be complex and require specialized knowledge [20].

4. Conclusion

When evaluating a patient with a suspected neurological disorder, the age at onset of symptoms is an important factor to consider. If the patient has a baseline developmental delay, the age at onset of neurological symptoms or regression is regarded as the age of onset.

It is useful to classify neurological disorders into broad groups based on the age at onset. For example, infancy is typically defined as the period from 1 to 12 months of age, while the late infantile/early juvenile onset period is from 1 to 5 years of age. The early infantile, late infantile/early juvenile, and late childhood periods are from 0 to 2 years, 2 to 6 years, and 6 to 12 years, respectively.

This classification can help guide the diagnostic workup and management of the patient. For example, certain neurological disorders, such as infantile spasms, are more common in the early infantile period, while others, such as Rett syndrome, typically present in the late infantile/early juvenile period.

In addition to the age at onset, other factors such as the pattern of inheritance, family history, and clinical features can also help narrow down the differential diagnosis and guide the diagnostic workup. A thorough evaluation by a neurologist or other specialist is necessary to make an accurate diagnosis and develop an appropriate management plan.

Conflict of interest

The authors declare no conflict of interest.

Author details

Bita Shalbafan
Neurologist, Tehran, Iran

*Address all correspondence to: b-shalbafan@alumnus.tums.ac.ir

References

[1] International League against Epilepsy [Internet]. 2022. Available from: https://www.epilepsydiagnosis.org/syndrome/epilepsy-syndrome-groupoverview.html [Accessed: July 15, 2022]

[2] Bindu PS. Neurometabolic disorders: A diagnostic approach. Indian Journal of Practical Pediatrics. 2016

[3] Vanderver A. Tools for diagnosis of leukodystrophies and other disorders presenting with white matter disease. Current Neurology and Neuroscience Reports. 2005;**5**:110-118. DOI: 10.1007/s11910-005-0008-1. Available from: https://link.springer.com/article/10.1007/s11910-005-0008-1

[4] Pediatric Neurology Neurometabolic Disorders: A Diagnostic Approach. Available from: https://www.researchgate.net/publication/305622211_PEDIATRIC_NEUROLOGY_NEUROMETABOLIC_DISORDERS_A_DIAGNOSTIC_APPROACH [Accessed: May 06, 2023]

[5] Azarmina M, Shalbafan B. AI accuracy in Papilledema diagnosis in Fundus photographs within 201 eyes. Biomedical Journal of Science and Technology Research;**51**(2). DOI: 10.26717/BJSTR.2023.51.008086

[6] Christensen J. The epidemiology of posttraumatic epilepsy. Seminars in Neurology. 2015;**35**:218-222. Available from: https://www.thieme-connect.com/products/ejournals/pdf/10.1055/s-0035-1552923

[7] Chen BS, Meyer BI, Saindane AM, et al. Prevalence of incidentally detected signs of intracranial hypertension on magnetic resonance imaging and their association with papilledema. JAMA Neurology. 2021;**78**:718-725

[8] Sandhu MR, Mandel M, Mcgrath H, et al. Management of patients with medically intractable epilepsy and anterior temporal lobe encephaloceles. Journal of Neurosurgery. 2022;**136**:709-716

[9] Urbach H, Jamneala G, Mader I, et al. Temporal lobe epilepsy due to meningoencephaloceles into the greater sphenoid wing: A consequence of idiopathic intracranial hypertension. Neuroradiology. 2018;**60**:51-60

[10] Saavalainen T, Jutila L, Mervaala E, et al. Temporal anteroinferior encephalocele: an underrecognized etiology of temporal lobe epilepsy. Neurology. 2015;**85**:1467-1474

[11] Tse GT, Frydman AS, Shea MF, et al. Anterior temporal encephaloceles: Elusive, important, and rewarding to treat. Epilepsia. 2020;**61**:2675-2684

[12] Campbell ZM, Hyer JM, Lauzon S, et al. Detection and characteristics of temporal encephaloceles patients with refractory epilepsy. AJNR American Journal of Neuroradiology. 2018;**39**:1468-1472

[13] Martinez-Poles J, Toledano R, Jimenez-Huete A, et al. Epilepsy associated with temporal pole encephaloceles: An unrecognized manifestation of idiopathic intracranial hypertension. Clinical Neuroradiology. 2021;**31**:575-579

[14] Thottiyil JJ, Prasad A, Dutta DJ, Anand R, SA NSP, Nadarajah J, et al. Temporal lobe encephalocele with epilepsy in a young female: An atypical presentation of idiopathic intracranial hypertension. Neurology India. 2022;**70**:1618-1621

[15] Michael BD, Solomon T. Seizures and encephalitis: Clinical features, management, and potential pathophysiologic mechanisms. Epilepsia. 2012;**53**(Suppl. 4):63-71

[16] Bonello M. Infective causes of epilepsy. Seminars in Neurology. 2015;**35**:235-244 Available from: https://www.thieme-connect.com/products/ejournals/pdf/10.1055/s-0035-1552619

[17] Vogrig A, Gigli GL, Nilo A, Pauletto G, Valente M. Seizures, epilepsy, and NORSE secondary to autoimmune encephalitis: A practical guide for clinicians. Biomedicine. 2023;**11**:44. DOI: 10.3390/biomedicines11010044

[18] Jang Y, Kim DW, Yang KI, Byun JI, Seo JG, No YJ, et al. Clinical approach to autoimmune epilepsy. Journal of Clinical Neurology. 2020;**16**(4):519-529. DOI: 10.3988/jcn.2020.16.4.519

[19] Geis C, Planagumà J, Carreño M, Graus F, Dalmau J. Autoimmune seizures and epilepsy. The Journal of Clinical Investigation. 2019;**129**(3):926-940. DOI: 10.1172/JCI125178

[20] Levite M, Goldberg H. Autoimmune epilepsy – Novel multidisciplinary analysis, discoveries and insights. Frontier in Immunology. 2022;**12**:726. DOI: 10.3389/fimmu.2021.762743

[21] Husari KS, Dubey D. Autoimmune epilepsy. Neurotherapeutics. 2019;**16**(3):685-702. DOI: 10.1007/s13311-019-00750-3

Chapter 5

Childhood Absence Epilepsy

Luigi Vetri, Carola Costanza, Margherita Siciliano, Francesco Precenzano, Beatrice Gallai and Marco Carotenuto

Abstract

Childhood absence epilepsy (CAE) is a common epilepsy syndrome characterized by absence seizures affecting young children and representing 18% of all diagnosed cases of epilepsy in school-age children. Absence seizures are classically very frequent during the day and each seizure lasts a short time, from about 10 to 20 seconds, it ends abruptly, and awareness and responsiveness are severely impaired. The typical EEG pattern in CAE is a bilateral, synchronous, and symmetrical discharge of complex spike-wave rhythms at 3 Hz (range of 2.5–4 Hz), with sudden onset and termination. CAE is genetically determined, the mode of inheritance and genes involved remain not fully clarified but the final outcome is the dysregulation of cortico-thalamic-cortical circuit that plays a crucial role in the pathophysiology of absence seizures. CAE may have an impact on patients' lives in terms of negative consequences in neurocognitive and neuropsychological aspects that should always be considered during a global evaluation of a child with epilepsy.

Keywords: childhood absence epilepsy, absence, seizure, epilepsy, EEG

1. Introduction

Childhood absence epilepsy (CAE) is a common form of idiopathic generalized epilepsy of childhood, corresponding to 18% of all diagnosed cases of epilepsy in school-age children. CAE is characterized by multiple typical absence seizures, together with, on the electroencephalogram, synchronous and symmetrical bilateral discharges of 2.5–4 Hz generalized spike-waves [1].

In 2017, the International League Against Epilepsy (ILAE) classification [2] CAE was included in the group of idiopathic generalized epilepsy (IGE) together with juvenile absence epilepsy (JAE), juvenile myoclonic epilepsy (JME), and epilepsy with generalized tonic–clonic seizures alone (GTCA). In 2022, the Task Force on Nosology and Definitions defined IGE as a distinct subgroup of Genetic Generalized Epilepsies because they generally have a good prognosis, a polygenic inheritance, an overlap symptomatology, similar EEG findings, and they do not evolve in epileptic encephalopathy but can evolve into each other [3].

2. Epidemiology

CAE incidence is 6.3–8.0 cases per 100,000 per year [4], and it represents 18% of epilepsy in school-aged children. In a cohort study of children, the CAE prevalence was estimated between 0.4 and 0.7 per 1000 people [5]. CAE, with some exceptions, is more frequent in girls than in boys (75 vs. 60%) [6]. Usual CAE onset is between 4 and 10 years of age with a peak at 5–7 years [7].

3. Clinical presentation

CAE is characterized by frequent absence seizures, up to 100 daily seizures, in otherwise typically developmental children although comorbid neurodevelopmental disorders may be present [1, 8, 9]. The sudden loss of awareness is the essential characteristic of CAE absence seizures, with loss of contact with the surrounding environment, lack of response to calls, and psychomotor arrest [10].

Absence seizures are typically multiple during the day and can be often underrecognized.

Many children stop their activities, but some may continue to carry out their tasks in an impaired manner, and at the end of the seizure, there is an immediate return to normal activity [11]. Another important ictal-associated clinical feature consists of fixed gaze, regular eye movements at 3 Hz, and eyes opening in cases where they are initially closed [11]. Frequently, automatisms can be observed, especially in longer crises and during hyperventilation.

The automatisms are mostly oro-alimentary or gestural movements and are repeated in a similar way in the same child. In any case, these movements may not be present in all absence seizures even in the same child, and their presence is not influenced by age or state of vigilance [12].

Mild clonic and tonic movements may also be present during the first seconds of the absence seizure, while tonic drops are never mentioned. Pallor is also common.

Urine incontinence occurs in exceptional cases [13]. Furthermore, some studies report perioral myoclonus and arrhythmic and single myoclonic jerks of the limbs, head, or trunk present during seizures in some children [11, 14]. These are mostly retropulsive movements of the head [9].

The duration of seizures is influenced by various factors: induction (hyperventilation or intermittent light stimulation), the state of arousal, sleep deprivation, pharmacological treatment, and individual factors [12, 15]. The typical duration of absence seizure is 3–20 seconds; a seizure duration of less than 4 seconds or more than 30 seconds is not typical of CAE [7]. Generalized tonic–clonic may rarely occur in the period of a high frequency of seizures and sometimes during adolescence, they can underline the evolution to another IGE [16].

4. Electroencephalogram

The typical EEG pattern of CAE is a bilateral, synchronous, and symmetrical discharge of complex spike-wave rhythms at 3 Hz (range 2.5–4 Hz), with sudden onset and termination. Often, a recovery of function is observed towards the end of the crisis and sometimes functions can be spared **(Figure 1)** [10]. However, EEG discharges sometimes have maximum frontal amplitude or may exhibit initial unilateral focal spikes [17].

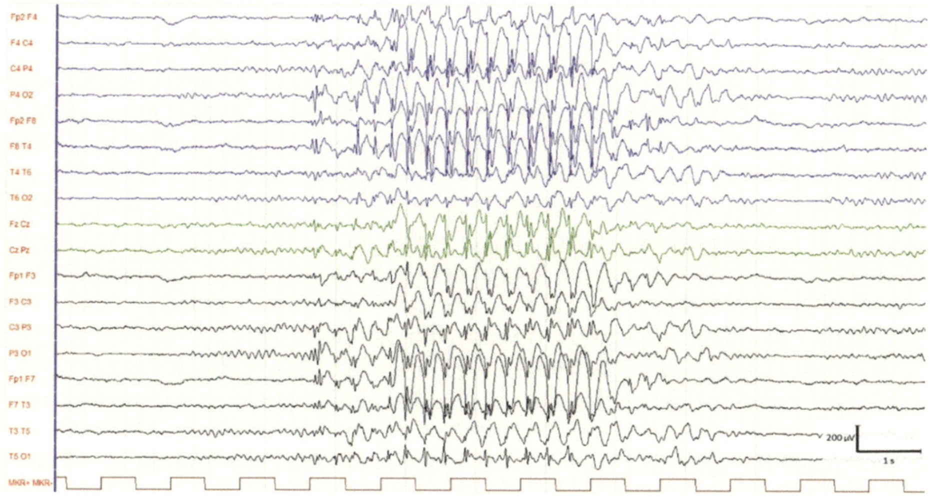

Figure 1.
EEG example of patient with CAE with typical 3 Hz spike and wave discharges.

Sadleir and colleagues meticulously described the electroclinical characteristics of absence seizures and analyzed videos of 339 absence seizures from a cohort of 47 children with a recent diagnosis of AIH. The authors demonstrated that the mean seizure duration was 9.4 seconds (ranging from 1 to 44 seconds), shorter than the 12.4 seconds previously reported. In 50% of CAE seizures, the initial generalized discharge is characterized by a typical spike-wave, while others are characterized by single spikes, polyspikes, or an atypical irregular generalized slow wave.

Seizures without a regular slow wave discharge are rare. The majority of discharges consist of spike-wave complexes with one or two spikes per wave. Children with photosensitivity are more likely to have three or four spikes per wave. The discharge may show a degree of variability at the end of the seizure, especially coinciding with drowsiness, sleep, or hyperventilation. In these circumstances, the regular ictal discharge can be interrupted by slow waves, complexes of different frequencies and/or morphology, or brief and transient interruptions of the ictal discharge [18].

Hyperventilation induces absence seizures in 83% of patients while intermittent light stimulation induces absence seizures in 21% of patients [11].

The interictal electroencephalographic activity of CAE is characterized by normal background activity but in 92% of cases, it is possible to document paroxysmal interictal activity consisting of bursts of generalized spike-wave discharges. However, focal epileptiform interictal discharges could be present not only in central areas but also in frontal, temporal, and parietal areas [11, 18].

Delta, rhythmic, intermittent occipital activity, also described as delta, rhythmic, bilateral, posterior activity is another interictal abnormality of CAE. This activity is characterized by rhythmic bursts at 2.5–4 Hz over the occipital regions, and it is enhanced by hyperventilation and drowsiness while attenuated by eye opening and deep sleep [11, 19]. The presence of multiple spikes (more than three), 3–4 Hz spike-wave paroxysms of less than 4 seconds, or segmentation of the ictal discharge are not typical of CAE and suggest a worse prognosis [7].

5. Pathophysiology of CAE

Theories on epileptogenesis. The mechanisms underlying the generalized spike-and-wave discharges of absence seizures have been analyzed in many studies, for more than 7 decades, but the debate continues [1]. Absence seizures evidently involve bilateral cortical and subcortical networks that are part of the default state system [20]. In 1941, Jasper and Kershman, analyzing the electroencephalograms of patients suffering from childhood petit mal, proposed a subcortical origin of absence seizures, imagining a thalamic pacemaker that projected simultaneously to both cerebral hemispheres. Subsequently, a second thalamo-cortical projection system was hypothesized to contribute to the spread of spike-wave discharges originating from the intralaminar nucleus of the thalamus [21].

These results led Jasper and Droogleever Fortujn, in 1947, to the first experimental model of spike-and-wave: the cat thalamic stimulation model. A stimulation of 3 cycles/sec in the intralaminar nucleus of the thalamus can produce a bilateral and synchronous 3 Hz spike-and-wave EEG discharge, associated with an absence-like behavioral modification [22].

In 1954, Penfield introduced the expression "centrencephalic epilepsy", to indicate the genesis in the trunk and diencephalon, responsible for the origin of generalized seizures with initial loss of consciousness and bilateral onset synchronous on the EEG [23].

In 1952, Gibbs and Gibbs questioned the centrencephalic theory, hypothesizing instead that a diffuse cortical process was at the origin of spike-and-wave discharges. Data in favor of these hypotheses were produced by administering proconvulsant substances via the arterial route: the intracarotid injection determined the appearance of bilateral and synchronous spike-and-wave -type EEG discharges; the same substances were ineffective when administered into the vertebral arteries. Further data in support of a cortical origin of the absences were obtained through depth recordings carried out in patients suffering from lesional epilepsy of the frontal lobe and generalized EEG anomalies [24]; the latter led Luders and Niedermeyer to formulate the hypothesis of a fronto-mesial origin of absences and, more generally, of idiopathic generalized epilepsies [25, 26].

At the end of the 1960s, Gloor proposed a reticulocortical mechanism, attributing an essential role to the genesis of bilateral and synchronous POs to both the cortex and the thalamus and trunk. The theory was based on the stimulation of the thalamus in the cat, capable of inducing PO discharges only after the application of penicillin in the cortex. This led to the belief that the factor necessary for the genesis of PO discharges was in the condition of cortical hyperexcitability [27, 28].

The intrathalamic network. In 1991, Buzsaki studied the thalamo-cortical system in a strain of rats with spontaneous PO discharges, hypothesizing a "thalamic clock", initially responsible for discharges, located in the thalamic reticular nucleus. In this nucleus, one would find the cells capable of triggering the recruitment of the intrathalamic network and the thalamo-cortical connections, at the basis of the origin of the physiological spindle figures.

PO discharges would be the result of an abnormal rhythmic oscillation of the intrathalamic network, which would impose its own rhythm on the cortex [29]. This theory, which revived the concept of "centrencephalic epilepsy", was subsequently supported by further studies on different strains of epileptic rats (GAERS, WAG, Rij). In these animals, both lesions to the reticular nucleus of the thalamus and deactivation of the cortex resulted in the disappearance of spontaneous PO discharges, demonstrating that both structures are necessary for the generation of absences [30].

In recent studies, the temporal relationships between thalamic and cortical structures during spike-and-wave discharges have been clarified with nonlinear signal analysis methods.

The result is evidence of a cortical "focus" at the level of the perioral region of the somato-sensory cortex, from which the discharges then propagate to other areas of the cortex, for example, to the thalamus [31].

Conversely, some studies have shown that the onset of spike-wave activity is in the thalamus [32, 33]. According to other researchers, these findings would be false representations of cortical activities occurring in sites distant from the typical focus of the somatosensory cortex [34].

Based on this conflicting evidence, the general consensus is that although some forms of spike-and-wave activity may originate from the cortex or thalamus, the entire thalamocortical circuit is required to generate typical spike-and-wave discharges [20].

In particular, one hypothesis is that the initiation of the discharge is induced by the cortex, and that the thalamic structures are subsequently responsible for its amplification and maintenance through the thalamo-cortical connections. In this way, the theory of the "cortical focus" underlying absence seizures appears to be a synthesis between the cortical and reticulocortical theories [34].

Today, the cortico-thalamic-cortical circuit is considered to play a crucial role in the pathophysiology of absence seizures. Neurons of the thalamic nucleus reticularis can fire in an oscillatory pattern or continuously in single spikes. Changes in the type of firing patterns depend on low-threshold transient calcium channels known as T-type channels neurons from the thalamic nucleus reticularis. After depolarization, T-type channels before becoming inactive allow a little calcium inflow. The reactivation of these channels requires a long hyperpolarization facilitated by GABA-B receptors. Therefore, T-type channel abnormalities or GABA-B hyperactivation can provoke abnormal oscillatory rhythms. Similarly, mutation in genes coding for T-type calcium channels and GABA receptors has been related to CAE etiopathogenesis [35].

6. EEG-fMRI studies

Associated EEG-fMRI studies have shown changes in activity in all components of the default state system [20, 31]. Many studies describe activation of the thalamus, as well as inactivation of the medial frontal cortex, medial parietal cortex, anterior and posterior cingulate cortex, lateral parietal cortex, and simultaneous activation-inactivation of the lateral frontal cortex [36–38].

Increased activity in the primary motor, somatosensory, visual and auditory cortex, and cerebellum are also reported on fMRI, while decreased activity is often observed in the basal ganglia and pons [36, 37, 39].

Only a few studies have attempted to relate fRMI in absence seizures to reduced behavioral performances [36, 37]: The results suggest widespread changes as behavior deteriorates. An important challenge appears to be represented by fMRI studies that simplify the analysis of hemodynamic response functions related to brain activity.

Time-course analyses have shown that an activation in fMRI begins in the medial frontal and parietal cortex 10 seconds before the onset of the absence seizure on the EEG [40, 41]. These early changes in fMRI are followed by complex sequences of activation and inactivation with different time courses in cortical and subcortical structures, most of which cannot be measured by standard hemodynamic functional responses used for conventional fMRI analysis [10].

Furthermore, new approaches are indispensable to detect these important fMRI changes that may be related to the deterioration of consciousness. All studies support the conclusion that spike-and-wave discharges are the result of epileptic activity generated within the cortico-thalamocortical circuit. Therefore, the EAI sticks to the definition of an epileptic system understood as a condition underlying a persistent susceptibility of the thalamic-cortical system, capable in its fullness of generating seizures. The epileptic system hypothesis postulates that the propensity to generate seizures depends on a specific susceptibility of a specific neural system to an epileptogenic factor.

Available data support the idea of a trigger zone within a specific area of the thalamo-cortical system that has a genetically determined epileptogenic susceptibility [1], a pretreatment topological disruption is present and primarily affects the prefrontal-thalamocortical circuit underlining that an alteration brain network topology and structural–functional connectivity is an intrinsic feature of CAE [42].

7. Spike and wave discharges pathophysiology

Spike and wave discharges are the electrographic hallmarks of CAE. On the intracellular microelectrode level, cortical neurons show depolarization coinciding with the spikes and hyperpolarization corresponding to the wave of the EEG spike-wave complexes. Very briefly, the rhythmicity of the spike-wave complexes is the consequence of intrathalamic and thalamo-cortical oscillatory electrical activity [43], which would be generated in genetically predisposed subjects [1].

Key components of this circuit include cortical pyramidal neurons, relay nuclei neurons of the thalamus, and the reticular nucleus of the thalamus [1]. The intrathalamic and thalamo-cortical oscillatory circuits would depend on the activation of transmembrane calcium currents, defined as transient T, on which the genesis, at the cortical level, of the rhythmic discharges of spike-wave complexes at 3 Hz would depend.

On a neurotransmitter level, the ideal condition for the genesis of these discharges is given by a high level of both glutamate-asparthaergic excitation and GABA A-mediated inhibition [44]. Furthermore, the role of GABA B receptors appears crucial at the level of the thalamic relay nuclei, the activation of which would facilitate the genesis of spike-wave discharges [43].

In particular, the main synaptic connections of the thalamic-cortical circuit include glutamatergic fibers extending from the neocortical pyramidal cells to the thalamic reticular nucleus (NRT) and GABAergic fibers extending from the thalamic reticular nucleus to the thalamic relay neurons. The cellular events that guarantee the maintenance of oscillatory rhythms are ensured by the presence of Ca ++ channels and T-Transient at the level of the neurons of the reticular nucleus of the thalamus (NRT) [1].

According to the cortical focus theory, spike-and-wave activity rapidly propagates through cortico-cortical networks from the cortical focus of origin. Oscillatory circuits of the thalamic-cortical network amplify and sustain discharges [45]. The origin of the ictal discharge is characterized by the activation of the dorsolateral frontal and orbital frontal regions [45].

8. Genetics

Although CAE is genetically determined, the mode of inheritance and genes involved remain not fully clarified. In most cases, CAE susceptibility is likely due to the influence of multiple genes and only a few genes confer a monogenic risk for CAE.

The calcium channel genes are associated with CAE especially CACNA1H and CACNG3 genes [46]. Also, GABA A and B receptor genes such as GABRG2, GABRA1, GABRB3, GABAB1, and GABAB2 genes have been implicated in the epileptogenesis of CAE [47]. Moreover, there is literature evidence of the involvement of chloride channels genes (CLCN2) as a susceptibility locus in CAE [48]. If there are atypical clinical features such as early onset, drug resistance, intellectual disability, and movement disorders, a glucose transporter 1 deficiency (SLC2A1 gene) should be suspected [49].

Mutations in patients with CAE were sometimes described in SLC2A1 gene coding for glucose transporter type 1 although the mutation rate in patients with CAE seems to be low [50].

Lastly, there are also recurrent CNVs that must be considered within the multiple possible genetic causes of CAE such as 15q11.2, 15q13.3, and 16p13.11 microdeletion [51].

9. Pharmacological treatment of CAE

The first-line antiseizure medications (ASMs) commonly used for CAE is ethosuximide (ETX), valid alternatives as initial treatment for CAE, valproic acid (VPA), and lamotrigine (LTG). VPA has more adverse effects, and LTG is less effective compared to ETX [52].

Topiramate, zonisamide, and levetiracetam [53–55] can be considered when other treatments fail.

Carbamazepine, oxcarbazepine, phenobarbital, phenytoin, tiagabine, and vigabatrin may worsen absence seizures or cause absence status epilepticus and should not be administered [56].

10. The evolution and prognosis of CAE

Studies on the evolution and prognosis of CAE are relatively incomplete due to the inaccuracy of diagnosis, definitions, and inclusion and exclusion criteria. Furthermore, the variability of the prognosis depends on the duration of follow-up [1]. CAE, if correctly recognized using correct diagnostic criteria recently revised in 2022 by ILAE (**Table 1**), has an excellent prognosis for seizure remission and for successful treatment with ASMs. The rate of remission cases reported in literature varies in the range of 56–84% [57, 58].

In a prospective study, Callenbach et al. observed that the total duration of epilepsy and the average age at the end of remission corresponded to 3.9 years and 9.5 years, respectively; the two criteria studied increased in children who presented seizures 6 months after enrollment. Few children, equal to 7%, of those who presented crises after 12–17 years of follow-up showed a good prognosis [57].

Retrospective studies highlight the possibility that patients in remission were under-reported and this contributed to an apparently lower remission rate. Grosso et al., however, demonstrated that the inclusion criteria had a notable influence on the outcomes of these results [59].

Patients were classified into two groups: the first with a diagnosis based on the ILAE classification and the second with a diagnosis established on more rigid diagnostic criteria proposed by Loiseau and Panayiotopoulos [7]. The second group showed a higher remission rate defined by the percentage of seizure-free patients in the absence of ASMs treatment for a period of ≥1 year (82 vs. 51%), a lower incidence

	Mandatory	Alerts*	Exclusionary
Seizures	Typical absence Seizures	GTCS prior to or during the peak of absence seizures seizures duration >30 s or with postictal confusion Absences rarely occur in untreated patients	Prominent myoclonic, Myoclonic–absence, or eyelid myoclonia seizures Presence of atonic, tonic, atypical absence, focal impaired awareness seizures
EEG	Synchronous and symmetrical discharge of complex spike-wave rhythms at 3 Hz (range 2.5–4 Hz). An ictal EEG is not required for diagnosis	Unilateral epileptiform discharges Lack of hyperventilation activation Recording a typical staring spell without EEG correlate Slowing of the EEG background	Diffuse background slowing
Age at onset	between 4 and 10 years, peak at 5–7 years	2–3 or 11–13 years	<2 or > 13 years
Development at onset	Normal	Mild intellectual disability	Moderate to profound intellectual disability
Neurological Exam	Normal	Potentially relevant neurological examination abnormalities, excluding incidental findings	
Imaging	Normal (An MRI is not required for diagnosis)	Potentially relevant abnormal neuroimaging, excluding incidental findings	

Source: Modified from Hirsch et al. [3].
Note: CAE, childhood absence epilepsy; CSF, cerebrospinal fluid; EEG, electroencephalogram; and GTCS, generalized tonic–clonic seizures.
**Alert criteria are absent in most CAE patients, but they may be rarely present. Alerts do not exclude CAE diagnosis but their presence should lead to a rethink of the diagnosis or to make further investigations.*

Table 1.
Diagnostic criteria for CAE.

of generalized tonic–clonic seizures (8 vs. 30%), and absence of relapse upon discontinuation of AEDs (0 vs. 22%).

The estimated percentage of patients developing generalized tonic–clonic seizures range from 8 to 69%, as can be seen from the literature [45, 57]. Most often, generalized tonic–clonic seizures occur 5–10 years after the onset of the absence seizure. Some patients develop a refractory syndrome known as juvenile myoclonic epilepsy [58]. However, all these observations relating to the evolution of the syndrome and/or the earlier onset of generalized tonic–clonic seizures remain controversial. Furthermore, the development of myoclonic seizures also suggests a worse prognosis. Other negative prognostic factors include: type of absence, late onset of absence seizures (after age 8), abnormal EEG background activity, multiple spikes, and presence of focal abnormalities [58, 59].

On the contrary, a favorable prognostic factor is the early remission of the seizure following the introduction of an appropriate antiepileptic treatment [60]. EEG abnormalities can persist even in adults and even in seizure-free subjects [1].

11. Differential diagnoses

Differential diagnosis includes other IGE syndromes. Epilepsy with myoclonic absences (EMA) is characterized by an alteration of contact with the environment of variable extent (from mild to complete); bilateral myoclonus (prevalent in the limbs) constitutes the constant characteristic of this type of crisis and is often associated with a tonic contracture, especially proximal. Seizures begin and end abruptly, and their duration varies from 10 to 60 seconds. The frequency is high and absences often occur 10 times a day; in 14% of cases, they can be induced by SLI or occur during slow sleep, awakening the patient. The interictal EEG is usually normal. In a third of cases, generalized PO sequences and rarer focal or multifocal PO bursts can be observed. The critical EEG is characterized by a discharge of bilateral, synchronous, and symmetric 3 Hz PO complexes. Polygraphic recordings document that myoclonias are closely correlated with the tips of the complex. The prognosis appears to be closely correlated with the presence of associated generalized tonic–clonic (CGTC) seizures (worse if present) [9].

The juvenile absence epilepsy (JEA) has the same characteristics as CAE, but the age of onset is pubertal (9–13 years), and its frequency is lower: 1–10 per day.

Seizures are often associated with CGTC and more rarely, with sporadic myoclonia. Absence-type status epilepticus (SE) is also described. The interictal EEG is normal or with short bursts or groups of PO and PPO. PO discharges, predominantly frontal, are generally faster than 3 Hz (3.5–4 Hz), the first complex is often faster, and PPOs are frequent. However, seems to be very difficult to exactly define a certain border between these CAE and JAE, and there always remains a gray area between the two syndromes [61].

However, studies relating to this syndromic group are few. In a video-EEG study, Panayiotopoulos et al. [62], reported the characteristics of the absence seizures of patients with EAG, compared to those typical of EAI: Contact breaking is less important, eyes opening during the absence is less common, crises last longer, and discharges can become fragmented [9].

Reflex absences. They are classified based on the stimulus capable of causing them. According to the ILAE classification, reflex syndromes can be caused by visual, proprioceptive, and somatosensory stimuli and there are seizures caused by music, reading, contact with hot water, etc. However, the ILAE specifically mentions only idiopathic photosensitive occipital epilepsy, primary reading epilepsy, and startle epilepsy as reflex epilepsies. Seizures are usually of a generalized type on a clinical level (absences, myoclonia, generalized tonic–clonic seizures) [9].

Juvenile myoclonic epilepsy is a syndrome that begins in the pubertal period (12–18 years) and is typically characterized by massive, bilateral, single, arrhythmic, irregular myoclonic seizures, predominant in upper limbs, without alteration of contact with the environment. Myoclonias are more frequent after waking up at night and cause objects to fall from the hands. In addition to myoclonic seizures, subjects present CGTC (preceded by myoclonic seizures) in 85% of cases and absence seizures in approximately a third of cases. The critical EEG is characterized by generalized bursts of PP at 10–16 Hz, of medium voltage, followed by short sequences of slow waves at 1–3 Hz. Absence seizures are short and generally not associated with automatisms and from an EEG point of view, they correlate with discharges of irregular PO and PPO complexes at 3–4 Hz (with inscriptions of components at 2–7 Hz). The interictal EEG is characterized by normal background activity, with the possibility of recording short groups of generalized and irregular PO and PPO complexes [1].

The epilepsy with eyelid myoclonia should be considered if there are rhythmic and fast (>4 Hz) jerks of the eyelids, with an upward deviation of the eyeballs and with possible subtle head extension; seizures can be very frequent and can be triggered by eye closure and photic stimulation [63].

12. Neurocognitive aspects in CAE

The impact of absence epilepsy on neurocognitive functions can vary widely. While some individuals may not experience significant cognitive difficulties, others may exhibit varying degrees of impairment in cognitive domains such as memory, attention, and executive functions.

Even in the absence of visible seizures (ictal events), individuals with absence epilepsy may exhibit abnormal electrical brain activity during interictal periods. These interictal discharges can disrupt cognitive processing and contribute to neurocognitive impairments [64].

Furthermore, cognitive difficulties may depend on cortical microdysplasias for example, on the characteristics of absence seizures themselves (aura, ictal phase, perictal phase) or on anticonvulsant pharmacological treatment [65].

In 2013, a double-blind randomized clinical trial conducted on 446 children affected by CAE showed a high rate of attention deficits in patients before treatments and even if seizures were well controlled. Despite average intellectual ability, 35% of untreated children demonstrated the presence of clinically significant attention problems. Attention deficits in children with CAE have an important impact on learning and achievement. Although children may become seizure-free with a normalized EEG, attention deficits persist even with the use of the most efficacious medication. Furthermore, in this study, valproic acid affects attention more than either lamotrigine or ethosuximide [66].

Various areas of cognitive domains may be compromised in CAE patients. Below, we will analyze some of the cognitive domains affected by alterations or impairment.

To explain CAE comorbidities, several studies have evaluated the intellectual functioning of affected subjects in relation to healthy patients or other types of epilepsy. For assessing cognitive problems in children, intelligence tests are considered a first-line instrument. The results of intelligence quotient (IQ) tests were largely analyzed in various studies. Despite being within the normal range, the average IQ scores in current studies were significantly lower than those in healthy controls [65, 67, 68]. IQ appeared to be related to the frequency and extent of seizures [69]. The common hypothesis in multiple studies is that IQ could reflect the impact of seizures, considering lower age of onset and not well-controlled seizures, as negatively affecting cognition and language skills [70, 71]. Lower IQs in CAE children [72] are even related to social difficulties and behavioral problems. Performance analysis by testing found lower IQ scores in CAE subjects compared to those with partial or generalized seizures.

There is some evidence that a reduction of sleep spindle density in N2 sleep phase can represent a good EEG marker in predicting cognitive impairment in children with CAE [73].

The study of ASMs role on cognition has been widely debated in CAEs. Some studies have reported a significantly beneficial effect of AEDs, through seizure control, on various cognitive functions such as motor fluidity, memory, and attention [74]. However, Nolan et al. in 2003 [70] showed that the use of more than two anticonvulsant drugs was associated with lower IQ scores.

Pavone et al. conducted a study on 16 children suffering from an epileptic syndrome defined by clear diagnostic criteria: epilepsy with absences. All patients had negative neuroimaging and were under pharmacological treatment with ethosuximide, valproate, or both [65]. The researchers excluded all children with generalized tonic–clonic seizures. The abilities of these patients were compared with a control group of the same number. The study showed that global cognitive abilities appeared average (with total IQ between 71 and 120), although significantly deficient compared to the control group.

Visuospatial skills were moderately deficient in subjects with absence seizures. Furthermore, a selective deficit in non-verbal memory was observed, while language functions were generally preserved.

Studies conducted on surface-based morphometry in CAE patients have shown that the average intellectual functioning of these children reflects the neuropathology underlying CAE and is linked to plasticity and reorganization of brain development. In fact, CAE patients did not have cortical morphometric measures in line with age or related to other variables such as age of onset, seizure frequency, or AED intake. In particular, an increase in sulcal depth was found at the level of the superior temporal gyrus, the somatosensory region, and the left frontal lobe [75]. This suggests widespread neurocognitive deficits in patients with absence seizures involving multiple brain systems.

Several studies investigating verbal IQ in children with CAE, such as those conducted by Jones et al., Caplan et al., or Henkin et al. [8, 76, 77] revealed worse performances than normal children especially in verbal fluency [78].

Children affected by absence epilepsy often experience attention-related problems [69].

During absence seizures, individuals often experience a sudden and temporary loss of awareness or consciousness. This means their attention to their surroundings, ongoing activities, and conversations are interrupted [79].

Attention appears particularly vulnerable to epileptic activity [80]. At the same time, seizures themselves are typically very brief (usually lasting only a few seconds), these interruptions can disrupt attention and concentration, especially if they occur frequently throughout the day [81].

A study by Cerminara et al. [82] assessed the attentional characteristics of children with CAE using tests that measure attention and discovered that patients with CAE had lower scores in the areas of vigilance, selective attention, and impulsivity compared to healthy controls.

Neuroimaging studies demonstrate significant changes in brain networks underlying attention, such as, for example, decreased activity in the anterior insula of the medial frontal cortex [1, 80].

Regarding how treatment affects attentional abilities, several studies agree that VPA can cause a worsening of attentional abilities more than other antiepileptic drugs [83].

Visual memory is impaired in children with CAE, as evidenced by multiple studies [75], while others have found no significant differences with children with other epileptic syndromes [84]. The presence of epileptic seizures in children and adolescents for several years can lead to problems with consolidating knowledge, which can negatively impact school results [85].

A deficit of executive functions is frequently found in subjects with epilepsy, as demonstrated by several studies [72, 84], even in CAE children compared to healthy controls [86]. The affected children showed difficulties in those domains of frontal executive functions such as decision-making skills, problem-solving, and planning, in particular, the difficulty they had concerned knowing how to change responses based on external requests.

13. Comorbidities

Studies focused on CAE have shown the presence of learning disabilities in this group of patients. Frequent absence seizures, if uncontrolled, can interfere with the learning process, particularly in school-aged children. These seizures can disrupt the continuity of lessons and affect the ability to retain information [8].

Vanasse et al., in a 2005 study [87], demonstrated that even children suffering from generalized seizures, specifically absence seizures, had difficulties in reading. Many children struggle to acquire the phonological strategies that underlie learning to read.

The involvement of both the temporal and frontal lobes in the phonological reading processes has largely been demonstrated; about this, patients with complex partial epilepsy show difficulties in reading skills [88, 89].

Despite seizures per se, duration, age of onset, and other factors influencing cognitive abilities, and variables such as familial factors or neuropsychological comorbidities are often significant in influencing underperformance at school in epileptic children [77].

Attention deficit hyperactivity disorder (ADHD) may co-occur with epilepsy in some cases, especially in children. The presence of both conditions can complicate diagnosis and management.

ADHD is the most common disorder in preschool and school-age children with epilepsy [90]. It has a negative impact on the quality of life and represents a significant risk factor for academic performance [91].

There is evidence pointing to a complex relationship between ADHD and seizure disorders. Some literature studies have demonstrated the presence of ADHD, anxiety, and depression disorders in children affected by CAE [8, 92]. A close association between these pathologies has recently been postulated. The mechanisms underlying attention deficits are still unknown and appear to be different between generalized and focal epilepsies [93].

ADHD and selective attention deficits are more prevalent in children with CAE than in typically developing children. ADHD is reported to be comorbid in children with childhood epilepsy in about 12–17% of cases [94]. In several studies, comorbid ADHD was diagnosed in about 40% of CAE patients [95, 96].

In particular, some findings suggest that recurrent seizures and treatment may not be the main etiological factor underlying ADHD [97] and that attention deficit and hyperactivity symptoms start before the diagnosis of epilepsy [95, 97]. From most recent studies, it is therefore clear that the early diagnosis of ADHD in comorbidity with epilepsy is useful to correctly plan a pharmacological treatment.

Furthermore, a significant proportion of patients affected by epilepsy, between 10 and 15%, manifests intellectual disability [65].

The comorbidity between intellectual disability and epilepsy is well-documented and relatively common. Studies have shown that individuals with intellectual disabilities have a higher risk of developing epilepsy than the general population. Individuals with intellectual disabilities may have a higher predisposition to epilepsy due to underlying structural brain abnormalities or genetic factors [98]. As discussed, epilepsy can potentially lead to intellectual impairment, particularly if seizures are frequent, severe, or difficult to control.

In this regard, for example, a syndrome has been described as a phenotype of the 15q13.3 microdeletion syndrome, characterised by absence seizures and intellectual disability [99].

Regarding behavioral problems, there is an ongoing debate as to whether these problems are an integral part of epilepsy syndrome or whether they develop due to factors associated with the disease [100].

Some researchers argue that behavioral problems are intrinsic to certain epilepsy syndromes. They believe that abnormal electrical activity in the brain during seizures or interictal periods can directly affect mood and behavior [101].

In addition, the resulting psychosocial disruption of diagnosis in patients' lifestyles or therapeutic interventions with AEDs can also cause behavioral effects [102]. Some AEDs may lead to mood swings, aggression, or other behavioral changes [103].

In this regard, we recall a 1997 study, in which Elaine et al. hypothesized that patients suffering from absence epilepsy could have more serious psychosocial disorders than patients suffering from chronic non-neurological pathologies [104].

In the study, two groups of patients were compared: one group was made up of young adults who had been diagnosed with CAE, and the other group was affected by juvenile rheumatoid arthritis. The study found that patients suffering from CAE had many more psychosocial problems than those suffering from arthritis. Patients with CAE, in fact, had greater scholastic difficulties, increased need for scholastic support, major behavioral problems, and relationship difficulties with peers and family members.

Psychiatric and emotional disorders were reported in both groups but were more common in subjects with CAE. Furthermore, remission of epileptic seizures did not lead to an improvement in the psychosocial condition, although subjects whose seizure remission was not observed showed a remarkable worsening and a higher risk of psychiatric and emotional disorders.

Furthermore, the presence of these comorbidities can contribute to causing difficulties in socialization and poor academic results in patients with CAE.

Individuals with epilepsy may also have comorbid psychiatric disorders, such as depression, anxiety, or ADHD [105]. At least 50–60% of patients with epilepsy develop psychiatric disturbances.

Depression is one of the most common psychiatric disorders in people with epilepsy. The physical and emotional impact of seizures, as well as the social stigma associated with epilepsy, can contribute to feelings of sadness and hopelessness [106].

Depressive and anxiety syndromes are the most frequent disorders in adults with epilepsy [107], and there is much literature evidence that epilepsy and depression share a bidirectional relationship, although the nature of this relationship remains unclear at present [108].

Anxiety disorders, including generalized anxiety disorders and specific phobias, are more prevalent in individuals with epilepsy. The unpredictability of seizures can lead to heightened anxiety [109, 110].

A study on 45 subjects with CAE and 41 healthy controls, between the ages of 6 and 16 years specifically examined anxiety and depression symptoms, revealing that children with CAE demonstrated higher rates of anxiety and depression symptoms and greater general psychosocial problems, while intractability, disease duration, and medication effects were not associated with higher rates of affective problems [99], although an iatrogenic role in this context cannot be ruled out.

However, Ott et al., in 2001 [111], administrating the Diagnostic Interview for the Evaluation of Psychopathological Disorders in Children and Adolescents (K-SADS-PL) reported mood disorders, specifically anxiety and depression disorders, in 12% of 48 children suffering from complex partial seizures and in 18% of 40 children suffering from CAE.

Caplan et al., in a 2005 study [92] conducted on 171 children, of which 100 with complex partial epilepsy, 71 with absence epilepsy, and 93 healthy children, demonstrated that 33% of children affected by complex partial epilepsy and absence epilepsy suffer from affective disorders, especially anxiety disorders. Individuals with epilepsy, particularly those with comorbid psychiatric disorders, may be at a higher risk of suicide [112].

In conclusion, we can state that although CAE is historically considered a benign disorder, children affected may present several difficulties in psychosocial adaptation [1].

An early diagnosis and evaluation of comorbidities can favor the implementation of specific interventions such as cognitive-behavioral therapy, school and educational approaches, and psychological support [1] that help to contain and reduce negative prognostic outcomes related to neurodevelopmental disorders.

14. Iatrogenic effects of treatment

Antiepileptic drugs (AEDs) are a common cause of cognitive and behavioral effects in children with CAE.

Cognitive functions, including vigilance, attention, psychomotor speed, memory, and mood, are also the domains affected. Despite iatrogenic effects, epilepsy treatment may positively affect patients' cognitive performances by stopping or decreasing seizures [113, 114].

Some common cognitive side effects associated with certain AEDs include memory problems, attention and concentration, language and verbal skills [114].

Certain AEDs may affect language abilities, leading to difficulties with speech or comprehension.

New antiepileptic drugs generally produce fewer cognitive effects, although topiramate may impair attention, memory, and language.

Most studies agree that high doses of antiepileptic drugs and polytherapy compromise concentration, motor skills, and memory functions [65].

The effects of valproate have not yet been carefully studied in children, but we know that the drug has mild effects on cognitive abilities [101, 115].

A more recent study reports that valproic acid does not cause consequences on cognitive abilities if the ammonia level is controlled [116] and that ethosuximide does not cause cognitive deterioration, although the available data are still sketchy [116].

In some cases, cognitive side effects may be dose-dependent, meaning that higher doses of medication are more likely to cause cognitive impairment [66].

A targeted therapy evaluating the benefits and potential side effects of AEDs is recommended, searching for the best way to control seizures with minimal cognitive side effects [102].

15. Conclusion

CAE is a common epilepsy syndrome whose diagnosis is not difficult, and it should be considered in every child with normal development and multiple daily absence seizures associated with 3 Hz generalized spike-and-wave. Seizures are usually drug-responsive, and it is possible to retain first-line monotherapies: ethosuximide followed by valproate. CAE may be associated with impairments in executive function, attention, and concentration, and it may be correlated with learning disabilities, language disorders, and neuropsychological problems such as anxiety and depression. According to this perspective, taking care of patients with CAE may require a multispecialty approach especially when it is necessary to treat cognitive-behavioral disorders or drug-resistant seizures.

Author details

Luigi Vetri[1,2], Carola Costanza[3*], Margherita Siciliano[2], Francesco Precenzano[2], Beatrice Gallai[4] and Marco Carotenuto[2]

1 Oasi Research Institute-IRCCS, Troina, Italy

2 Clinic of Child and Adolescent Neuropsychiatry, Department of Mental Health, Physical and Preventive Medicine, University of Campania "Luigi Vanvitelli", Caserta, Italy

3 Department of Sciences for Health Promotion and Mother and Child Care "G. D'Alessandro", University of Palermo, Palermo, Italy

4 Department of Surgical and Biomedical Sciences, University of Perugia, Perugia, Italy

*Address all correspondence to: ccostanza@oasi.en.it; marco.carotenuto@unicampania.it

References

[1] Matricardi S, Verrotti A, Chiarelli F, Cerminara C, Curatolo P. Current advances in childhood absence epilepsy. Pediatric Neurology. 2014;**50**(3):205-212

[2] Scheffer IE, Berkovic S, Capovilla G, Connolly MB, French J, Guilhoto L, et al. ILAE classification of the epilepsies: Position paper of the ILAE Commission for Classification and Terminology. Epilepsia. 2017;**58**(4):512-521

[3] Hirsch E, French J, Scheffer IE, Bogacz A, Alsaadi T, Sperling MR, et al. ILAE definition of the idiopathic generalized epilepsy syndromes: Position statement by the ILAE task force on nosology and definitions. Epilepsia. 2022;**63**(6):1475-1499

[4] Loiseau J, Loiseau P, Guyot M, Duche B, Dartigues JF, Aublet B. Survey of seizure disorders in the French southwest. I. Incidence of epileptic syndromes. Epilepsia. 1990;**31**(4):391-396

[5] Jallon P, Latour P. Epidemiology of idiopathic generalized epilepsies. Epilepsia. 2005;**46**:10-14

[6] Waaler PE, Blom BH, Skeidsvoll H, Mykletum A. Prevalence, classification, and severity of epilepsy in children in western Norway. Epilepsia. 2000;**41**(7):802-810

[7] Panayiotopoulos CP. Syndromes of idiopathic generalized epilepsies not recognized by the international league against epilepsy. Epilepsia. 2005;**46**:57-66

[8] Caplan R, Siddarth P, Stahl L, Lanphier E, Vona P, Gurbani S, et al. Childhood absence epilepsy: Behavioral, cognitive, and linguistic comorbidities. Epilepsia. 2008;**49**(11):1838-1846

[9] Mecarelli O. Manuale teorico pratico di elettroencefalografia. Wolters Kluwer Health. Springer Healthcare Italy Srl; 2009

[10] Blumenfeld H. Impaired consciousness in epilepsy. The Lancet Neurology. 2012;**11**(9):814-826

[11] Sadleir LG, Farrell K, Smith S, Connolly MB, Scheffer IE. Electroclinical features of absence seizures in childhood absence epilepsy. Neurology. 2006;**67**(3):413-418

[12] Sadleir LG, Scheffer IE, Smith S, Carstensen B, Farrell K, Connolly MB. EEG features of absence seizures in idiopathic generalized epilepsy: Impact of syndrome, age, and state. Epilepsia. 2009;**50**(6):1572-1578

[13] Hirsch E. Childhood absence epilepsy and related syndrome. Epileptic Syndromes in Infancy, Childhood and Adolescence. Montrogue: John Libbey Eurotext; 2005:315-335

[14] Sadleir LG, Farrell K, Smith S, Connolly MB, Scheffer IE. Electroclinical features of absence seizures in sleep. Epilepsy Research. 2011;**93**(2-3):216-220

[15] Sadleir LG, Scheffer IE, Smith S, Carstensen B, Carlin J, Connolly MB, et al. Factors influencing clinical features of absence seizures. Epilepsia. 2008;**49**(12):2100-2107

[16] Ma X, Zhang Y, Yang Z, Liu X, Sun H, Qin J, et al. Childhood absence epilepsy: Elctroclinical features and diagnostic criteria. Brain Dev. 2011;**33**(2):114-119

[17] Unterberger I, Trinka E, Kaplan PW, Walser G, Luef G, Bauer G. Generalized

nonmotor (absence) seizures—What do absence, generalized, and nonmotor mean? Epilepsia. 2018;**59**(3):523-529

[18] Seneviratne U, Cook M, D'Souza W. The electroencephalogram of idiopathic generalized epilepsy. Epilepsia. 2012;**53**(2):234-248

[19] Seneviratne U, Cook M, D'Souza W. The prognosis of idiopathic generalized epilepsy. Epilepsia. 2012;**53**(12):2079-2090

[20] Blumenfeld H. Cellular and network mechanisms of spike-wave seizures. Epilepsia. 2005;**46**:21-33

[21] Jasper H, Kershman J. Electroencephalographic classification of the epilepsies. Archives of Neurology and Psychiatry. 1941;**45**(6):903-943

[22] Jasper HH. Expreimental studies on the functional anatomy of petit mal epilepsy. Research Publications – Association for Research in Nervous and Mental Disease. 1947;**26**:272-298

[23] Penfield W. Epileptic automatism and the centrencephalic integrating system. Research publications-Association for Research in Nervous and Mental Disease. 1952;**30**:513-528

[24] Gibbs FA, Gibbs EL. Atlas of Elec-Troencephalography. Cambridge, Mass: Addi-son. Wesley Press, Inc; 1950

[25] Luders H, Lesser RP, Dinner DS, Morris HH. Generalized epilepsies: A review. Cleveland Clinic Quarterly. 1984;**51**(2):205-226

[26] Niedermeyer E. The generalized epilepsies: A clinical electroencephalographical study. Springfield, Ill: Charles C Thomas Publisher; 1972

[27] Gloor P. Generalized Cortico-reticular epilepsies some considerations on the pathophysiology of generalized bilaterally synchronous spike and wave discharge. Epilepsia. 1968;**9**(3):249-263

[28] Gloor P. Neurophysiological basis of generalized seizures termed centrencephalic. The Physiopathogenesis of the Epilepsies. Springfield, Ill: Charles C Thomas Publisher; 1969:209-236

[29] Buzsáki G. The thalamic clock: Emergent network properties. Neuroscience. 1991;**41**(2-3):351-364

[30] Coenen AML, Van Luijtelaar E. Genetic animal models for absence epilepsy: A review of the WAG/Rij strain of rats. Behavior Genetics. 2003;**33**:635-655

[31] Meeren HKM, Pijn JPM, Van Luijtelaar ELJM, Coenen AML, da Silva FHL. Cortical focus drives widespread corticothalamic networks during spontaneous absence seizures in rats. Journal of Neuroscience. 2002;**22**(4):1480-1495

[32] Inoue M, Duysens J, Vossen JMH, Coenen AML. Thalamic multiple-unit activity underlying spike-wave discharges in anesthetized rats. Brain Research. 1993;**612**(1-2):35-40

[33] Seidenbecher T, Staak R, Pape HC. Relations between cortical and thalamic cellular activities during absence seizures in rats. European Journal of Neuroscience. 1998;**10**(3):1103-1112

[34] Meeren H, van Luijtelaar G, da Silva FL, Coenen A. Evolving concepts on the pathophysiology of absence seizures: The cortical focus theory. Archives of Neurology. 2005;**62**(3):371-376

[35] Hu B, Guo D, Wang Q. Control of absence seizures induced by the pathways

connected to SRN in corticothalamic system. Cognitive Neurodynamics. 2015;**9**:279-289

[36] Berman R, Negishi M, Vestal M, Spann M, Chung MH, Bai X, et al. Simultaneous EEG, fMRI, and behavior in typical childhood absence seizures. Epilepsia. 2010;**51**(10):2011-2022

[37] Gotman J, Grova C, Bagshaw A, Kobayashi E, Aghakhani Y, Dubeau F. Generalized epileptic discharges show thalamocortical activation and suspension of the default state of the brain. National Academy of Sciences of the United States of America. 2005;**102**(42):15236-15240

[38] Moeller F, LeVan P, Muhle H, Stephani U, Dubeau F, Siniatchkin M, et al. Absence seizures: Individual patterns revealed by EEG-fMRI. Epilepsia. 2010;**51**(10):2000-2010

[39] Moeller F, Siebner HR, Wolff S, Muhle H, Granert O, Jansen O, et al. Simultaneous EEG-fMRI in drug-naive children with newly diagnosed absence epilepsy. Epilepsia. 2008;**49**(9):1510-1519

[40] Benuzzi F, Mirandola L, Pugnaghi M, Farinelli V, Tassinari CA, Capovilla G, et al. Increased cortical BOLD signal anticipates generalized spike and wave discharges in adolescents and adults with idiopathic generalized epilepsies. Epilepsia. 2012;**53**(4):622-630

[41] Carney PW, Masterton RAJ, Harvey AS, Scheffer IE, Berkovic SF, Jackson GD. The core network in absence epilepsy: Differences in cortical and thalamic BOLD response. Neurology. 2010;**75**(10):904-911

[42] Yang T, Ren J, Zhang Y, Zhang T, Zhou H, Yang M, et al. Pretreatment topological disruptions of whole-brain networks exist in childhood absence epilepsy: A resting-state EEG-fMRI study. Epilepsy Research. 2022;**182**:106909

[43] Bergamini L, Bergamasco B, Mutani R. Manuale di Neurologia Clinica [Manual of Clinical Neurology]. Turin, Italy: Cortina; 2001

[44] Gloor P, Fariello RG. Generalized epilepsy: Some of its cellular mechanisms differ from those of focal epilepsy. Trends in Neurosciences. 1988;**11**(2):63-68

[45] Holmes MD, Brown M, Tucker DM. Are "generalized" seizures truly generalized? Evidence of localized mesial frontal and frontopolar discharges in absence. Epilepsia. 2004;**45**(12):1568-1579

[46] Liang J, Zhang Y, Chen Y, Wang J, Pan H, Wu H, et al. Common polymorphisms in the CACNA1H gene associated with childhood absence epilepsy in Chinese Han population. Annals of Human Genetics. 2007;**71**(3):325-335

[47] Thakran S, Guin D, Singh P, Singh P, Kukal S, Rawat C, et al. Genetic landscape of common epilepsies: Advancing towards precision in treatment. International Journal of Molecular Sciences. 2020;**21**(20):7784

[48] Everett K, Chioza B, Aicardi J, Aschauer H, Brouwer O, Callenbach P, et al. Linkage and mutational analysis of CLCN2 in childhood absence epilepsy. Epilepsy Research. 2007;**75**(2-3):145-153

[49] Arsov T, Mullen SA, Rogers S, Phillips AM, Lawrence KM, Damiano JA, et al. Glucose transporter 1 deficiency in the idiopathic generalized epilepsies. Annals of Neurology. 2012;**72**(5):807-815

[50] Koch H, Weber YG. The glucose transporter type 1 (Glut1) syndromes. Epilepsy & Behavior. 2019;**91**:90-93

[51] de Kovel CGF, Trucks H, Helbig I, Mefford HC, Baker C, Leu C, et al. Recurrent microdeletions at 15q11. 2 and 16p13. 11 predispose to idiopathic generalized epilepsies. Brain. 2010;**133**(1):23-32

[52] Kessler SK, McGinnis E. A practical guide to treatment of childhood absence epilepsy. Pediatric Drugs. 2019;**21**:15-24

[53] Piña-Garza JE, Schwarzman L, Wiegand F, Hulihan J. A pilot study of topiramate in childhood absence epilepsy. Acta Neurologica Scandinavica. 2011;**123**(1):54-59

[54] Verrotti A, Cerminara C, Domizio S, Mohn A, Franzoni E, Coppola G, et al. Levetiracetam in absence epilepsy. Developmental Medicine & Child Neurology. 2008;**50**(11):850-853

[55] Wilfong A, Schultz R. Zonisamide for absence seizures. Epilepsy Research. 2005;**64**(1-2):31-34

[56] Somerville ER. Some treatments cause seizure aggravation in idiopathic epilepsies (especially absence epilepsy). Epilepsia. 2009;**50**:31-36

[57] Callenbach PMC, Bouma PAD, Geerts AT, Arts WFM, Stroink H, Peeters EAJ, et al. Long-term outcome of childhood absence epilepsy: Dutch study of epilepsy in childhood. Epilepsy Research. 2009;**83**(2-3):249-256

[58] Wirrell EC, Camfield CS, Camfield PR, Gordon KE, Dooley JM. Long-term prognosis of typical childhood absence epilepsy: Remission or progression to juvenile myoclonic epilepsy. Neurology. 1996;**47**(4):912-918

[59] Grosso S, Galimberti D, Vezzosi P, Farnetani M, Di Bartolo RM, Bazzotti S, et al. Childhood absence epilepsy: Evolution and prognostic factors. Epilepsia. 2005;**46**(11):1796-1801

[60] Glauser TA, Holland K, O'Brien VP, Keddache M, Martin LJ, Clark PO, et al. Pharmacogenetics of antiepileptic drug efficacy in childhood absence epilepsy. Annals of Neurology. 2017;**81**(3):444-453

[61] Asadi-Pooya AA, Farazdaghi M. Childhood vs. juvenile absence epilepsy: How to make a diagnosis. Seizure. 2022;**102**:125-128

[62] Panayiotopoulos CP, Obeid T, Waheed G. Differentiation of typical absence seizures in epileptic syndromes. A video EEG study of 224 seizures in 20 patients. Brain. 1989;**112**(Pt 4):1039-1056. DOI: 10.1093/brain/112.4.1039

[63] Zawar I, Knight EP. Epilepsy with eyelid Myoclonia (Jeavons syndrome). Pediatric Neurology. 2021;**121**:75-80

[64] Verrotti A, Matricardi S, Rinaldi VE, Prezioso G, Coppola G. Neuropsychological impairment in childhood absence epilepsy: Review of the literature. Journal of the Neurological Sciences. 2015;**359**(1-2):59-66

[65] Pavone P, Bianchini R, Trifiletti RR, Incorpora G, Pavone A, Parano E. Neuropsychological assessment in children with absence epilepsy. Neurology. 2001;**56**(8):1047-1051

[66] Masur D, Shinnar S, Cnaan A, Shinnar RC, Clark P, Wang J, et al. Pretreatment cognitive deficits and treatment effects on attention in childhood absence epilepsy. Neurology. 2013;**81**(18):1572-1580

[67] Caplan R, Levitt J, Siddarth P, Wu KN, Gurbani S, Sankar R, et al. Frontal and temporal volumes in childhood absence epilepsy. Epilepsia. 2009;**50**(11):2466-2472

[68] Caplan R, Guthrie D, Komo S, Siddarth P, Chayasirisobhon S, Kornblum H, et al. Social communication in children with epilepsy. Journal of Child Psychology and Psychiatry. 2002;**43**(2):245-253

[69] Vega C, Vestal M, DeSalvo M, Berman R, Chung M, Blumenfeld H, et al. Differentiation of attention-related problems in childhood absence epilepsy. Epilepsy & Behavior. 2010;**19**(1):82-85

[70] Nolan MA, Redoblado MA, Lah S, Sabaz M, Lawson JA, Cunningham AM, et al. Intelligence in childhood epilepsy syndromes. Epilepsy Research. 2003;**53**(1-2):139-150

[71] Nolan MA, Redoblado MA, Lah S, Sabaz M, Lawson JA, Cunningham AM, et al. Memory function in childhood epilepsy syndromes. Journal of Paediatrics and Child Health. 2004;**40**(1-2):20-27

[72] Hermann BP, Jones JE, Sheth R, Koehn M, Becker T, Fine J, et al. Growing up with epilepsy: A two-year investigation of cognitive development in children with new onset epilepsy. Epilepsia. 2008;**49**(11):1847-1858

[73] Zhang W, Xin M, Song G, Liang J. Childhood absence epilepsy patients with cognitive impairment have decreased sleep spindle density. Sleep Medicine. 2023;**103**:89-97

[74] Siren A, Kylliäinen A, Tenhunen M, Hirvonen K, Riita T, Koivikko M. Beneficial effects of antiepileptic medication on absence seizures and cognitive functioning in children. Epilepsy & Behavior. 2007;**11**(1):85-91

[75] Tosun D, Siddarth P, Toga AW, Hermann B, Caplan R. Effects of childhood absence epilepsy on associations between regional cortical morphometry and aging and cognitive abilities. Human Brain Mapping. 2011;**32**(4):580-591

[76] Henkin Y, Sadeh M, Kivity S, Shabtai E, Kishon-Rabin L, Gadoth N. Cognitive function in idiopathic generalized epilepsy of childhood. Developmental Medicine and Child Neurology. 2005;**47**(2):126-132

[77] Jones JE, Siddarth P, Gurbani S, ShieldsWD,CaplanR.Cognition,academic achievement, language, and psychopathology in pediatric chronic epilepsy: Short-term outcomes. Epilepsy & Behavior. 2010;**18**(3):211-217

[78] D'Agati E, Cerminara C, Casarelli L, Pitzianti M, Curatolo P. Attention and executive functions profile in childhood absence epilepsy. Brain and Development. 2012;**34**(10):812-817

[79] Tenney JR, Glauser TA. The current state of absence epilepsy: Can we have your attention? The current state of absence epilepsy. Epilepsy Currents. 2013;**13**(3):135-140

[80] Killory BD, Bai X, Negishi M, Vega C, Spann MN, Vestal M, et al. Impaired attention and network connectivity in childhood absence epilepsy. NeuroImage. 2011;**56**(4):2209-2217

[81] Sánchez-Carpintero R, Neville BGR. Attentional ability in children with epilepsy. Epilepsia. 2003;**44**(10):1340-1349

[82] Cerminara C, D'Agati E, Casarelli L, Kaunzinger I, Lange KW, Pitzianti M, et al. Attention impairment in childhood absence epilepsy: An impulsivity problem? Epilepsy & Behavior. 2013;**27**(2):337-341

[83] Glauser TA, Cnaan A, Shinnar S, Hirtz DG, Dlugos D, Masur D, et al.

Ethosuximide, valproic acid, and lamotrigine in childhood absence epilepsy. New England Journal of Medicine. 2010;**362**(9):790-799

[84] Kernan CL, Asarnow R, Siddarth P, Gurbani S, Lanphier EK, Sankar R, et al. Neurocognitive profiles in children with epilepsy. Epilepsia. 2012;**53**(12):2156-2163

[85] Lopes AF, Monteiro JP, Fonseca MJ, Robalo C, Simões MR. Memory functioning in children with epilepsy: Frontal lobe epilepsy, childhood absence epilepsy, and benign epilepsy with centrotemporal spikes. Behavioural Neurology. 2014;**2014**:218637. DOI: 10.1155/2014/218637 [Epub 2014 Aug 3]. PMID: 25157201; PMCID: PMC4137508

[86] Conant LL, Wilfong A, Inglese C, Schwarte A. Dysfunction of executive and related processes in childhood absence epilepsy. Epilepsy & Behavior. 2010;**18**(4):414-423

[87] Vanasse CM, Béland R, Carmant L, Lassonde M. Impact of childhood epilepsy on reading and phonological processing abilities. Epilepsy & Behavior. 2005;7(2):288-296

[88] Black KC, Hynd GW. Epilepsy in the school aged child: Cognitive-behavioral characteristics and effects on academic performance. School Psychology Quarterly. 1995;**10**(4):345

[89] Mitchell WG, Chavez JM, Lee H, Guzman BL. Academic underachievement in children with epilepsy. Journal of Child Neurology. 1991;**6**(1):65-72

[90] Thome-Souza S, Kuczynski E, Assumpção F Jr, Rzezak P, Fuentes D, Fiore L, et al. Which factors may play a pivotal role on determining the type of psychiatric disorder in children and adolescents with epilepsy? Epilepsy & Behavior. 2004;**5**(6):988-994

[91] Fastenau PS, Shen J, Dunn DW, Austin JK. Academic underachievement among children with epilepsy: Proportion exceeding psychometric criteria for learning disability and associated risk factors. Journal of Learning Disabilities. 2008;**41**(3):195-207

[92] Caplan R, Siddarth P, Gurbani S, Hanson R, Sankar R, Shields WD. Depression and anxiety disorders in pediatric epilepsy. Epilepsia. 2005;**46**(5):720-730

[93] Steer CR. Managing attention deficit/hyperactivity disorder: Unmet needs and future directions. Archives of Disease in Childhood. 2005;**90**(suppl 1):i19-i25

[94] Reilly CJ. Attention deficit hyperactivity disorder (ADHD) in childhood epilepsy. Research in Developmental Disabilities. 2011;**32**(3):883-893

[95] Hermann B, Jones J, Dabbs K, Allen CA, Sheth R, Fine J, et al. The frequency, complications and aetiology of ADHD in new onset paediatric epilepsy. Brain. 2007;**130**(12):3135-3148

[96] Lee H-J, Kim E-H, Yum M-S, Ko T-S, Kim H-W. Attention profiles in childhood absence epilepsy compared with attention-deficit/hyperactivity disorder. Brain and Development. 2018;**40**(2):94-99

[97] Parisi P, Moavero R, Verrotti A, Curatolo P. Attention deficit hyperactivity disorder in children with epilepsy. Brain and Development. 2010;**32**(1):10-16

[98] Malone TJ, Kaczmarek LK. The role of altered translation in intellectual disability and epilepsy. Progress in Neurobiology. 2022;**213**:102267

[99] Muhle H, Mefford HC, Obermeier T, von Spiczak S, Eichler EE, Stephani U, et al. Absence seizures with intellectual disability as a phenotype of the 15q13.

3 microdeletion syndrome. Epilepsia. 2011;**52**(12):e194-e1e8

[100] Austin JK, Dunn DW. Progressive behavioral changes in children with epilepsy. Progress in Brain Research. 2002;**135**:419-427

[101] Aldenkamp AP, Arends J. Effects of epileptiform EEG discharges on cognitive function: Is the concept of "transient cognitive impairment" still valid? Epilepsy & Behavior. 2004;**5**:25-34

[102] Motamedi G, Meador K. Epilepsy and cognition. Epilepsy & Behavior. 2003;**4**:25-38

[103] Besag FMC. Behavioural effects of the newer antiepileptic drugs: An update. Expert Opinion on Drug Safety. 2004;**3**(1):1-8

[104] Wirrell EC, Camfield CS, Camfield PR, Dooley JM, Gordon KE, Smith B. Long-term psychosocial outcome in typical absence epilepsy: Sometimes a wolf in sheeps' clothing. Archives of Pediatrics & Adolescent Medicine. 1997;**151**(2):152-158

[105] Marsh L, Rao V. Psychiatric complications in patients with epilepsy: A review. Epilepsy Research. 2002;**49**(1):11-33

[106] Kanner AM, Balabanov A. Depression and epilepsy: How closely related are they? Neurology. 2002;**58** (8 suppl. 5):S27-S39

[107] Jacoby A, Baker GA, Steen N, Potts P, Chadwick DW. The clinical course of epilepsy and its psychosocial correlates: Findings from a UK community study. Epilepsia. 1996;**37**(2):148-161

[108] Bølling-Ladegaard E, Dreier JW, Kessing LV, Budtz-Jørgensen E, Lolk K, Christensen J. Directionality of the association between epilepsy and depression: A nationwide register-based cohort study. Neurology. 2023;**100**(9):e932-ee42

[109] Thapar A, Kerr M, Harold G. Stress, anxiety, depression, and epilepsy: Investigating the relationship between psychological factors and seizures. Epilepsy & Behavior. 2009;**14**(1):134-140

[110] Vega C, Guo J, Killory B, Danielson N, Vestal M, Berman R, et al. Symptoms of anxiety and depression in childhood absence epilepsy. Epilepsia. 2011;**52**(8):e70-ee4

[111] Ott D, Caplan R, Guthrie D, Siddarth P, Komo S, Shields WD, et al. Measures of psychopathology in children with complex partial seizures and primary generalized epilepsy with absence. Journal of the American Academy of Child & Adolescent Psychiatry. 2001;**40**(8):907-914

[112] Blumer D, Montouris G, Davies K, Wyler A, Phillips B, Hermann B. Suicide in epilepsy: Psychopathology, pathogenesis, and prevention. Epilepsy & Behavior. 2002;**3**(3):232-241

[113] Drane DL, Meador KJ. Cognitive and behavioral effects of antiepileptic drugs. Epilepsy & Behavior. 2002;**3**(5):49-53

[114] Meador KJ, Gilliam FG, Kanner AM, Pellock JM. Cognitive and behavioral effects of antiepileptic drugs. Epilepsy & Behavior. 2001;**2**(4):SS1-SS17

[115] Legarda SB, Booth MP, Fennell EB, Maria BL. Altered cognitive functioning in children with idiopathic epilepsy receiving valproate monotherapy. Journal of Child Neurology. 1996;**11**(4):321-330

[116] Ijff DM, Aldenkamp AP. Cognitive side-effects of antiepileptic drugs in children. Handbook of Clinical Neurology. 2013;**111**:707-718

Chapter 6

Perspective Chapter: VNS Nerve Stimulation in Epilepsy through Lifespan

Isabella D'Andrea-Meira

Abstract

Vagus nerve stimulation (VNS) has emerged as a significant therapeutic intervention for individuals with drug-resistant epilepsy (DRE) throughout their lifespan. DRE is a debilitating condition characterized by recurrent seizures that do not respond to traditional antiepileptic drugs, imposing substantial physical, cognitive, and emotional burdens on patients. VNS involves the implantation of a device that delivers electrical impulses to the vagus nerve, a major nerve connecting the brain to various organs. The mechanism of action is complex and not yet fully understood, but VNS has been found to modulate abnormal electrical activity in the brain, reducing the frequency and severity of seizures. This non-pharmacological approach offers a valuable alternative for patients who have exhausted conventional treatment options, improves their quality of life, and provides hope for seizure control. Importantly, VNS has demonstrated efficacy across different age groups, from children to adults, making it suitable for lifelong management of DRE. Furthermore, long-term studies have shown sustained benefits and safety of VNS, with potential positive effects on cognitive function and mood regulation. As a result, VNS represents a promising adjunctive therapy that can significantly impact the lives of individuals with drug-resistant epilepsy, offering them renewed hope and the potential for a better future.

Keywords: epilepsy, vagus nerve stimulation, neuromodulation, drug resistant epilepsy, network

1. Introduction

Epilepsy is a neurological disorder characterized by a persistent tendency to generate epileptic seizures [1]. Epilepsy manifests with a variety of symptoms, ranging from temporary confusion and loss of awareness to convulsions and unconsciousness.

While most patients achieve seizure control with antiseizure medications (ASMs), approximately 30% of individuals experience drug-resistant epilepsy (DRE), defined as failure of adequate trials of two tolerated, appropriately chosen, and used ASMs schedules to achieve seizure freedom [2–4]. It significantly impacts patients' daily lives, cognitive function, and psychosocial well-being. Managing DRE requires a multidisciplinary approach to address the diverse underlying etiologies and provide individualized treatment plans.

Surgical intervention has gained recognition as an effective alternative for individuals with pharmacoresistant epilepsy and is often considered when drug therapy fails to control seizures adequately. The goal is providing a chance for improved seizure control and enhanced quality of life [5, 6].

While surgical interventions have shown promising results, they may not be suitable for everyone. Non-surgical treatments offer alternatives for individuals who are not candidates for surgery or prefer less invasive approaches. One such non-surgical option is vagus nerve stimulation (VNS), which involves implanting a device that delivers electrical impulses to the vagus nerve, a major nerve in the neck. VNS can help reduce seizure frequency and intensity, although it may not eliminate seizures entirely [7].

Vagus nerve stimulation (VNS) is a non-pharmacological therapy that has been approved for the treatment of refractory epilepsy. The purpose of this chapter is to review the current literature on the use of VNS for the treatment of epilepsy and to discuss its mechanism of action, efficacy, and safety along lifespan.

2. Vagus nerve stimulation

VNS is a non-pharmacological treatment option, making it suitable for individuals who may not respond well to medications or are unable to tolerate their side effects. It can also be used in conjunction with medication, maximizing the chances of seizure control and improving overall outcomes for people with epilepsy.

In recent years, technological advancements have further improved the effectiveness and convenience of VNS therapy [8]. Newer devices offer increased customization and programming options, allowing healthcare providers to tailor treatment to each patient's unique requirements [9]. Additionally, some VNS devices are equipped with responsive neurostimulation capabilities, meaning they can detect and respond to the early signs of seizures, potentially aborting them before they manifest [9].

2.1 The Vagus nerve

The vagus nerve is the longest cranial nerve, originating from the brainstem and extending down to the abdomen. It is composed of both motor and sensory fibers, which allow it to carry signals in two directions: from the brain to different organs (motor function) and from organs back to the brain (sensory function) [10].

The vagus nerve's sensory fibers carry important information from the visceral organs back to the brain. These sensory signals help maintain homeostasis, allowing the brain to monitor and regulate various physiological processes.

In the vagus nerve, there are three main types of fibers: A fibers, B fibers, and C fibers. These fiber types differ in their diameter, conduction velocity, and the type of information they transmit. It's important to note that while A fibers and B fibers are myelinated and transmit signals relatively quickly, it is in these fibers that the VNS acts preferentially. C fibers are unmyelinated and conduct signals more slowly.

2.2 VNS and epilepsy history

The use of electrical stimulation for therapeutic purposes dates back to the ancient Greeks, who used electrical eels to treat headache and gout. In the modern era, the first application of electrical stimulation for therapeutic purposes was in the 18th century, when Benjamin Franklin used electricity to treat paralysis resulting from stroke [11].

The first documented attempt to use electrical stimulation for epilepsy was made in the late 19th century by English neurologist John Hughlings Jackson. He experimented with electrical stimulation of the vagus nerve to observe its impact on seizures [12]. It wasn't until the late 20th century that VNS gained significant traction as a viable treatment option for epilepsy. In the 1980s, researchers started investigating the therapeutic potential of VNS in animal models, which showed promising results in reducing seizure activity [13, 14].

The use of VNS specifically for epilepsy was first reported in the 1980s when a team of researchers at the University of Alabama in Birmingham implanted a VNS device in a patient with refractory epilepsy [15]. The patient experienced a significant reduction in the frequency and severity of seizures, and subsequent studies confirmed the device's efficacy in reducing seizure frequency in patients with refractory epilepsy [16].

Thereafter, prospective randomized clinical trials were carried out, and approval for use in patients with refractory epilepsy occurred in 1994 and 1997 in Europe and the United States, respectively [17]. Approval by ANVISA (National Health Surveillance Agency) for use in Brazil occurred in 2000. Recently, the neuromodulation committee of the Brazilian League of Epilepsy published recommendations for the use of the vagus nerve stimulator and stimulation deep brain [18].

The development of VNS devices has undergone significant improvements since the first clinical trials in the 1980s. The first-generation VNS device, developed by Cyberonics Inc., was implanted in the chest and connected to the vagus nerve via a lead wire. This device delivered fixed-frequency stimulation and required frequent adjustments to optimize therapeutic effects. Over the years, advancements in technology have led to the development of more advanced VNS devices. These newer devices allow for better customization of stimulation parameters and offer improved patient comfort and convenience.

Since then, VNS has been increasingly used as an adjunctive treatment for individuals with epilepsy, particularly those who do not respond well to medication. The therapy has demonstrated efficacy in reducing seizure frequency, improving quality of life, and providing an alternative option for patients who may not be suitable candidates for other forms of epilepsy surgery [7, 19].

In recent years, VNS has also shown potential for the treatment of other neurological and psychiatric conditions, such as depression and anxiety disorders. Ongoing research continues to explore the full range of therapeutic applications and optimize the effectiveness of VNS as a treatment option.

2.3 VNS mechanism of action

The mechanism of action of VNS is complex and not fully understood, but it is thought to involve a combination of effects on the central nervous system (CNS), autonomic nervous system (ANS), and immune system.

The afferent fibers of the vagus nerve transmit signals from the body to the CNS, providing sensory information about various physiological processes. The efferent fibers of the vagus nerve, on the other hand, transmit signals from the CNS to various organs and tissues in the body, regulating their function. The vagus nerve plays an important role in regulating many physiological processes, including heart rate, blood pressure, respiration, digestion, and immune function.

The mechanism of action of VNS involves various pathways, including the locus ceruleus, solitary tract, raphe nuclei, and cortical areas. The vagus nerve projects to various regions of the cerebral cortex, including the prefrontal cortex. Activation of the vagus nerve through VNS can lead to increased cortical excitability and the modulation of neural networks involved in cognition and emotional processing.

The locus ceruleus receives direct projections from the vagus nerve and is densely innervated by its fibers. This suggests that the locus ceruleus is a key player in mediating the effects of VNS on epilepsy [20]. The activation of the vagus nerve during VNS leads to the stimulation of the locus ceruleus, triggering a cascade of events that may contribute to its therapeutic effects [20, 21]. One of the major neurotransmitters released by the locus ceruleus is norepinephrine [22]. Norepinephrine has been shown to have both antiepileptic and proconvulsant properties, depending on the specific brain region and receptor subtype involved.

Furthermore, the locus ceruleus is interconnected with other brain regions implicated in epilepsy, such as the hippocampus and the cortex [23]. These connections allow for the integration of signals from the locus ceruleus with the broader epileptic network. Through its projections, the locus ceruleus can influence the excitability of these regions, potentially dampening epileptic activity. So, it contributes to the overall modulation of neuronal excitability and seizure activity by modulating the activity of inhibitory and excitatory neurotransmitters, as well as interacting with key brain regions involved in epilepsy.

Regarding neurotransmitters, studies have shown that VNS can modulate the release of neurotransmitters such as gamma-aminobutyric acid (GABA) and glutamate, which play critical roles in regulating neuronal excitability and seizure activity [24]. By increasing GABAergic inhibition and decreasing glutamatergic excitability, VNS helps to restore the balance of neurotransmission, thereby reducing the likelihood of seizures.

VNS has been found to influence EEG synchrony in individuals with epilepsy. Abnormal EEG synchrony, characterized by excessive synchronization or desynchronization, is often observed in epilepsy. VNS has been reported to modulate this abnormal synchrony and promote more balanced and coordinated neural activity. The exact mechanisms through which VNS achieves this effect are not yet fully understood, but it is thought to involve the modulation of neurotransmitters and neural networks involved in seizure generation [25, 26].

VNS has been shown to have modulatory effects on brain metabolism, particularly in regions associated with mood regulation, cognition, and seizure control. It is believed that VNS influences brain metabolism through its impact on neurotransmitter systems, neuroplasticity, and the autonomic nervous system. VNS has been shown to affect brain metabolism through its impact on cerebral blood flow and glucose utilization [27–29]. Research studies using neuroimaging techniques have demonstrated that VNS can increase regional cerebral blood flow and enhance glucose uptake in certain brain regions involved in seizure generation and propagation. This increased metabolic activity in these regions may promote the normalization of neuronal function and decrease seizure activity.

Finally, VNS is thought to modulate the immune system, which plays an important role in many physiological processes, including inflammation, wound healing, and tissue repair. VNS has been shown to reduce inflammation in animal models of arthritis and other inflammatory conditions, suggesting that it may have therapeutic potential for these conditions [30, 31].

Neuroplasticity is also important in seizure control. The proteome of postsynaptic density (PSD) is a protein complex located in the postsynaptic membrane, responsible for the structure, function, and plasticity of excitatory synapses in the central nervous system. It also known that neuronal activity regulates the protein composition of PSD. Researchers identified increased these protein content due to VNS showing the contribution to the plasticity of excitatory synapses [32].

The mechanism of action of VNS is intricate and not yet comprehensively understood. However, it is believed to involve a combination of influences on the central nervous system (CNS), autonomic nervous system (ANS), and immune system. To completely understand the mechanisms underlying the therapeutic effects of VNS, further research is required.

2.4 VNS surgical technique

I will describe a general overview of the surgical technique; please note that specific details and variations may exist depending on the patient, surgeon, and the device being used.

Here is a general description of the surgical technique for implanting a vagus nerve stimulation device:

2.4.1 Preoperative preparation

Before the surgery, the patient is typically evaluated and prepared for the procedure. This may involve conducting preoperative tests, reviewing the patient's medical history, and discussing any potential risks or complications.

2.4.2 Anesthesia

The surgery is usually performed under general anesthesia, ensuring that the patient is unconscious and does not feel any pain during the procedure.

2.4.3 Incision

The surgeon makes a small incision, typically on the left side of the chest, just below the collarbone. The exact location of the incision may vary based on the surgeon's preference and the patient's anatomy (**Figure 1**).

2.4.4 Pocket creation

A small pocket is created under the skin to hold the VNS device. This pocket is usually made in the upper chest area, but it can also be placed in the abdomen if necessary.

2.4.5 Lead placement

The surgeon carefully dissects down to the vagus nerve, usually located in the neck area. Two small electrodes, or leads, are wrapped around the vagus nerve. One lead is placed closer to the brainstem, while the other is positioned closer to the chest (**Figures 2** and **3**).

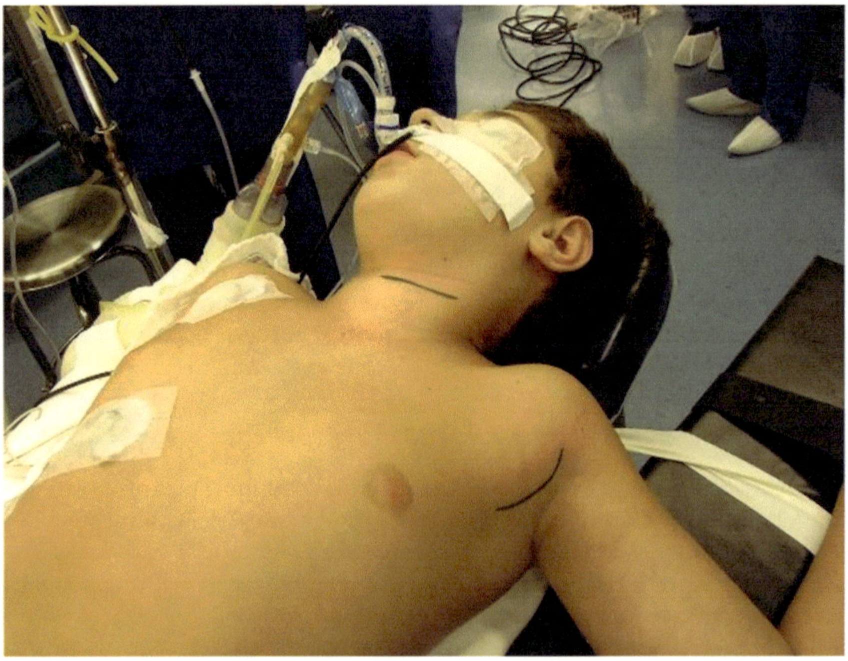

Figure 1.
Description of the cervical and thoracic incision.

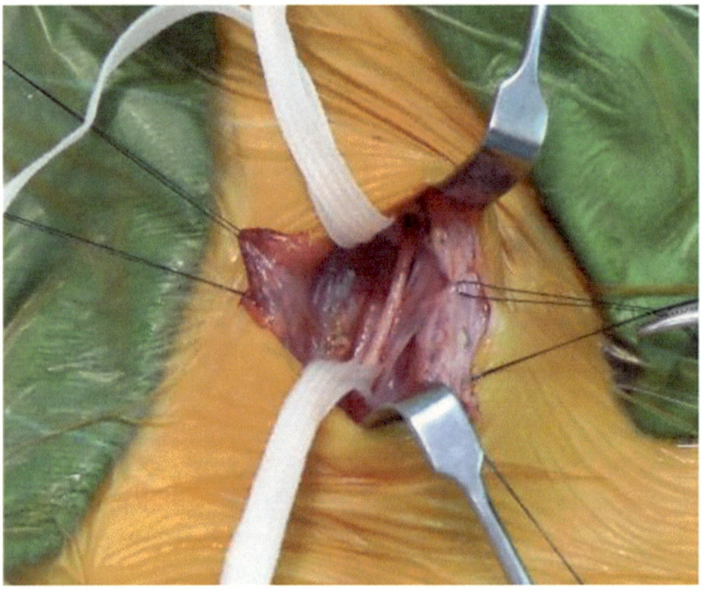

Figure 2.
Vagus nerve exposure.

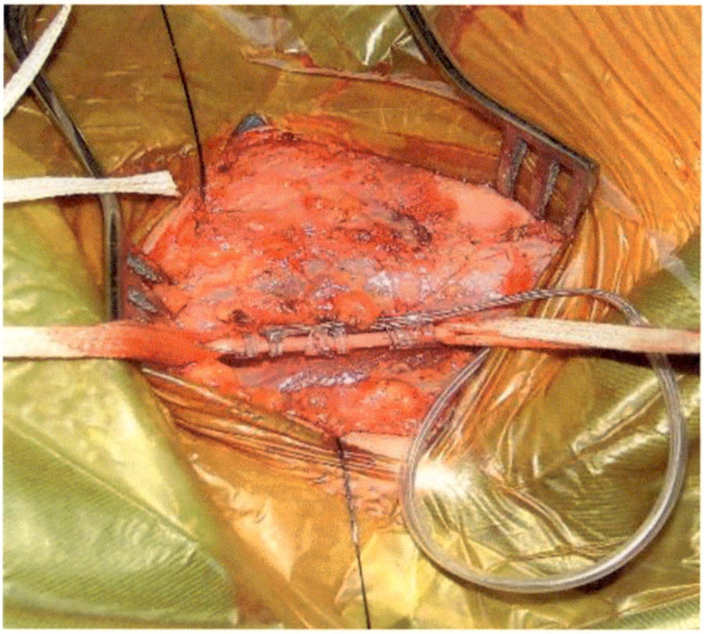

Figure 3.
Lead placement.

2.4.6 Tunneling

The leads are then tunneled beneath the skin from the neck area to the pocket created in the chest. The surgeon uses specialized instruments to carefully guide the leads to the desired location.

2.4.7 Connection

The leads are connected to the VNS device, which is placed in the pocket. The device is usually about the size of a silver dollar and contains a battery, electronics, and programming capabilities.

2.4.8 Closure

The incision is closed using sutures or surgical staples, and a sterile dressing is applied to the wound site.

2.4.9 Programming

After the surgery, the VNS device needs to be programmed to deliver the appropriate electrical impulses. This is typically done during a follow-up visit, using a handheld programming device that communicates with the implanted device.

It's important to note that VNS surgery carries certain risks and potential complications, including infection, bleeding, vocal cord dysfunction, device malfunction, and side effects related to nerve stimulation. The patient will be closely monitored after the procedure, and postoperative care instructions will be provided to aid in the healing process.

The specific details of the surgical technique may vary based on the patient's individual circumstances, the surgeon's expertise, and the specific VNS device being used.

3. Efficacy and safety through lifespan

3.1 VNS and children

Epilepsy affects people of all ages, including children. Despite pharmacological treatment, a significant proportion of pediatric patients continue to experience seizures and suffer from the adverse effects of medication. In such cases, alternative treatment options like vagus nerve stimulation (VNS) have emerged as a viable option.

3.1.1 Seizure reduction

VNS has demonstrated efficacy in reducing seizure frequency and intensity in children with epilepsy. Several clinical trials and observational studies have reported a significant reduction in seizure frequency by approximately 50% or more in a substantial proportion of pediatric patients [33–35].

Epilepsy has a complex etiology, and while it can be caused by a variety of factors, including brain injury, infections, or tumors, genetics play a significant role in the development of certain types of epilepsy. Advances in genetic research have led to the identification of numerous genes associated with various epilepsy syndromes. Research on the efficacy of VNS in genetic etiologies is still relatively limited, but several studies have explored its potential benefits in specific conditions.

Vagus nerve stimulation (VNS) has been the subject of investigation for several monogenic disorders, including Rett syndrome, Angelman syndrome, and Dravet syndrome. Initial research indicates that VNS could potentially improve respiratory function, heart rate variability, and overall behavioral functioning in individuals with these disorders [36, 37]. In the case of Angelman syndrome, researchers have reported improvements in communication skills, behavior [38].

Regarding Dravet syndrome, VNS has been investigated as an adjunctive treatment option, and studies have reported a reduction in seizure frequency and severity, as well as improvements in overall quality of life and cognitive function [39, 40]. In tuberous sclerosis, VNS is one of the therapeutic options that has shown promising efficacy in the management of seizures associated with tuberous sclerosis [41, 42].

VNS has been shown to provide sustained seizure reduction over an extended period. Studies have reported a decrease in seizure frequency even after several years of VNS therapy, with some patients experiencing complete seizure control [43–45].

In conclusion, VNS has demonstrated efficacy in reducing seizures and improving quality of life among children. It provides an additional treatment option for those who have refractory epilepsy and may not respond to traditional antiseizure medications. However, the response to VNS therapy can vary, and careful evaluation and consideration of individual cases are necessary. A collaborative approach involving medical professionals experienced in DRE is crucial in determining the most appropriate treatment plan for each patient.

3.1.2 Safety

When it comes to the safety of VNS in children, it's important to note that research and clinical experience in this area are more limited compared to adults. Nevertheless, several studies and clinical trials have been conducted to evaluate the safety and effectiveness of VNS in pediatric patients.

Overall, the available evidence suggests that VNS is generally safe for use in children. The most common side effects reported include hoarseness of voice, cough, throat pain, and difficulty swallowing, which are usually mild and transient. These side effects are believed to be related to the stimulation of the vagus nerve and the muscles of the larynx [44, 46–48].

Ongoing monitoring and follow-up care are essential to ensure the safety and effectiveness of VNS in children. Regular visits to the healthcare provider will allow for the assessment of any potential side effects or complications and adjustments to the stimulation parameters if needed.

3.2 VNs and adults

3.2.1 Seizure reduction

The use of VNS in adults has been used for decades since the first clinical trials. VNS therapy has shown effectiveness in reducing the frequency, severity, and duration of seizures. Research and clinical studies have provided evidence of seizure reduction in adults undergoing VNS therapy [49, 50]. The reduction in seizure frequency varies from person to person, and some individuals experience significant seizure reduction, while others may experience more modest improvements. It is important to note that VNS therapy does not guarantee complete seizure freedom but aims to decrease seizure frequency and improve quality of life.

In most published studies, the response rates for implantable VNS vary between 45% and 65% [51, 52]. Kawai et al. observed a median reduction in seizures of 25.0%, 40.9%, 53.3%, 60.0%, and 66.2% at 3, 6, 12, 24, and 36 months, respectively [52].

Over time, the benefits of VNS therapy may become more pronounced. Initially, the stimulation parameters may be adjusted to find the optimal settings for each individual, and it can take several months or longer to observe the full benefits of treatment. The response rate tends to improve over time significantly between the second and fifth year [53]. These observations could be related to neuroplasticity with neosynaptogenesis, as shown by Cramer et al. [54].

Overall, VNS therapy has demonstrated its potential to reduce seizure frequency and improve the quality of life for adults with epilepsy. However, it is important to consider the eligibility, discuss potential risks and benefits, and determine if it is an appropriate treatment option for their specific condition.

3.2.2 Safety

The implantation procedure carries some inherent risks, including infection, bleeding, and potential damage to surrounding structures. However, these risks are relatively low and can be minimized through proper surgical techniques and postoperative care [51].

The VNS device itself may cause some side effects or complications. These can include hoarseness or voice changes, coughing, shortness of breath, tingling or prickling in the skin, neck pain, and headache. However, many of these side effects are temporary and tend to diminish over time [49].

Regarding sleep disorders, VNS has the potential to alter breathing patterns and potentially lead to more episodes of apnea or hypopnea [55]. This effect appears to be more pronounced during periods when the VNS device is active; however, it can occur during OFF periods [56].

3.3 VNS and elderly

While the use of VNS in the elderly population is generally considered safe, there is limited research specifically focused on its efficacy in this age group.

3.3.1 Seizure reduction

The evidence for VNS efficacy in elderly individuals is not as extensive. Studies have shown that VNS can lead to a reduction in seizure frequency in elderly patients with epilepsy [57]. While the specific seizure reduction rates may vary, research indicates that a significant proportion of elderly individuals experience a reduction in seizure frequency by at least 50% [57].

3.3.2 Tolerability and safety

VNS has generally been found to be well-tolerated and safe in the elderly population. Adverse effects are typically mild and transient, including hoarseness, coughing, and shortness of breath. Serious complications are rare but can occur, such as infection or stimulation-related adverse events [57].

3.3.3 Potential cognitive benefits

Some studies have suggested that VNS may have cognitive benefits for elderly patients with epilepsy, including improvements in memory and executive functions. However, further research is needed to establish a clearer understanding of the cognitive effects of VNS in this population [58–60].

4. Dosing

Programming a VNS device involves setting parameters such as the stimulation strength, pulse width, frequency, and duty cycle to optimize seizure control. Here's a description of how to program VNS for epilepsy, including setting the duty cycle:

4.1 Setting stimulation strength

This initial programming session typically takes place a few weeks after the VNS device implantation surgery, allowing for recovery and healing.

Stimulation strength refers to the intensity of the electrical pulses delivered to the vagus nerve. It is usually measured in milliamperes (mA). Typically, we should start with a conservative stimulation strength and gradually increase it over time to achieve optimal seizure control while minimizing side effects.

According to clinical studies, the initial current should start with 0.25 and gradually increase by 0.25 at each visit until reaching the response dose. A computational study showed that a current of 1.75 to 2.0 should be enough to activate all vagus nerve fibers [61]. Specifically, the population-level target output current for VNS therapy is recommended to be set at 1.625 mA [62]. Patients who are gradually adjusted to output currents close to the desired level of 1.61 mA tend to experience fewer adverse events related to stimulation compared to those who are adjusted to higher or lower levels. Therefore, when determining the ideal dosage for individual patients, the primary factor to consider should be the output current. However, it's crucial to acknowledge that certain patients may require VNS output currents that deviate from the target level established for the general population, based on their specific circumstances.

4.2 Adjusting pulse width and frequency

Pulse width refers to the duration of each electrical pulse delivered by the VNS device, usually measured in microseconds (μs). A typical range for pulse width is 130–500 μs. However, biophysical data and modeling further support the use of pulse widths at or below 250 milliseconds, with lower pulse widths requiring an increase in the selected output current [62].

Frequency refers to the number of pulses delivered per second, measured in Hertz (Hz). Common frequencies range from 20 Hz to 30 Hz. Regarding the frequency of VNS therapy, there is currently insufficient robust data to advocate for the use of frequencies other than 20, 25, or 30 Hz in epilepsy to maximize clinical response. Therefore, these frequencies should be considered as the primary options [62].

Generally, these parameters are more related to the management of adverse effects. However, they may also influence the effectiveness of seizure control.

4.3 Configuring duty cycle

Duty cycle refers to the proportion of time the VNS device is actively stimulating versus the total time. It is usually expressed as a percentage. The duty cycle can be adjusted to modify the amount of stimulation delivered by the device.

A higher duty cycle means the device is actively stimulating for a larger proportion of time, which may provide increased seizure control but may also increase side effects. Conversely, a lower duty cycle means the device is stimulating for a smaller proportion of time, potentially reducing side effects but potentially compromising seizure control.

The optimal duty cycle for everyone varies, and finding the right balance often requires iterative adjustments during follow-up appointments with the healthcare professional.

There is still no robust evidence relating working time to types of seizures or response to VNS, which should be individualized for each patient.

4.4 Magnet and AutoStim

The VNS magnet is a handheld device that enables patients to deliver additional electrical stimulation to the vagus nerve when needed. It consists of a small magnet that can be placed over the implanted VNS device, triggering an immediate and short-term increase in stimulation. The VNS magnet offers patients the ability to self-manage their symptoms and provides a sense of control over their treatment.

Parameters	Visit 1	Visit 2	Visit 3	Visit 4	Visit 5	Visit 6	Visit 7	Visit 8
Output (mA)	0.25	0.50	0.75	1.0	1.25	1.5	1.5	1.5
Frequency (Hz)	20/30	20/30	20/30	20/30	20/30	20/30	20/30	20/30
Pulse width (μs)	250/500	250/500	250/500	250/500	250/500	250/500	250/500	250/500
Time ON (s)	30	30	30	30	30	30	30	30
Time OFF (min)	5	5	5	5	5	5	3	1.8

Table 1.
A step-by-step guide to programming vagus nerve stimulation.

When the VNS magnet is placed over the implanted VNS device, it activates a magnet switch within the device, leading to an increase in electrical stimulation. This temporary augmentation of vagus nerve activity can help alleviate acute symptoms or enhance therapeutic effects. The magnet switch is designed to ensure patient safety by limiting the duration and intensity of the additional stimulation. So, VNS magnet can be used during seizure events to provide immediate supplementary stimulation, potentially aborting or reducing the intensity of seizures.

Autostimulation is a feature integrated into some VNS devices that enables automatic adjustment of stimulation parameters based on real-time monitoring of heart frequency. By continuously monitoring heart rate, the VNS device can autonomously modulate the stimulation parameters, optimizing therapy delivery without requiring direct patient intervention [63].

Lo et al. showed the added effectiveness of AutoStim in children undergoing VNS treatment. Seizure reduction showed a substantial improvement, increasing from 60 to 83% after replacing the battery with AutoStim. When categorizing the results using the McHugh classification, the percentage of children achieving class I and II outcomes (≥50% seizure reduction) rose from 70 to 90% [64].

The table below shows the suggested evolution of parameters according to visits (**Table 1**).

In summary, the available evidence supports the adoption of current manufacturer dosing recommendations for VNS therapy in epilepsy. Output current is a crucial consideration when determining the optimal dose for individual patients. Further research is needed to explore the relationship between time-to-dose and time-to-response, as well as the impact of dose adjustments in non-responsive and over-responsive patients. Careful consideration of both efficacy and side effects is necessary when determining the parameters for VNS therapy in clinical practice.

5. Conclusion

The use of VNS in the management of epilepsy throughout an individual's lifespan offers significant benefits and has proven to be an effective treatment option. From early childhood to adulthood and into old age, VNS has shown promise in reducing seizure frequency and improving overall quality of life for individuals with epilepsy.

In children, VNS has been found to significantly decrease the number of seizures, allowing for better cognitive development and academic performance. It can also lead to a reduction in medication dosages and side effects, enhancing the child's overall well-being.

During adolescence and adulthood, VNS continues to be a valuable adjunctive treatment for epilepsy. It can provide seizure control, reduce seizure intensity, and lessen the need for rescue medications. Moreover, VNS has shown potential in improving mood and reducing comorbidities such as depression and anxiety, which are often associated with epilepsy.

As individuals with epilepsy age, VNS remains a viable option for seizure management. It has demonstrated long-term efficacy and safety, helping to maintain seizure control and reduce the risk of injury that can arise from seizures. Additionally, VNS offers the advantage of being adjustable and adaptable to changing seizure patterns over time, allowing for personalized treatment.

In conclusion, VNS is a valuable treatment option for epilepsy across the lifespan. Its ability to provide long-term seizure control, reduce medication dosages and side effects, improve mood, and adapt to changing seizure patterns makes it a valuable adjunctive therapy. Further research and advancements in VNS technology will likely continue to enhance its effectiveness and expand its potential benefits for individuals living with epilepsy.

Conflict of interest

The authors declare no conflict of interest.

Author details

Isabella D'Andrea-Meira
Paulo Niemeyer State Brain Institute, Rio de Janeiro, Brazil

*Address all correspondence to: sadandrea@yahoo.com.br

References

[1] Fisher RS, Acevedo C, Arzimanoglou A, Bogacz A, Cross JH, Elger CE, et al. ILAE official report: A practical clinical definition of epilepsy. Epilepsia. 2014;**55**:475-482. DOI: 10.1111/EPI.12550/SUPPINFO

[2] Brodie MJ, Barry SJE, Bamagous GA, Norrie JD, Kwan P. Patterns of treatment response in newly diagnosed epilepsy. Neurology. 2012;**78**:1548-1554. DOI: 10.1212/WNL.0b013e3182563b19

[3] Kwan P, Brodie MJ. Early identification of refractory epilepsy. New England Journal of Medicine. 2000;**342**:314-319. DOI: 10.1056/NEJM200002033420503

[4] Kwan P, Arzimanoglou A, Berg AT, Brodie MJ, Hauser WA, Mathern G, et al. Definition of drug resistant epilepsy: Consensus proposal by the ad hoc task force of the ILAE commission on therapeutic strategies. Epilepsia. 2010;**51**:1069-1077. DOI: 10.1111/J.1528-1167.2009.02397.X

[5] Wiebe S, Blume WT, Girvin JP, Liasziw ME. A randomized , controlled trial of surgery. The New England Journal of Medicine. 2008;**345**:311-318

[6] Téllez-Zenteno JF, Ronquillo LH, Moien-Afshari F, Wiebe S. Surgical outcomes in lesional and non-lesional epilepsy: A systematic review and meta-analysis. Epilepsy Research. 2010;**89**:310-318. DOI: 10.1016/j.eplepsyres.2010.02.007

[7] Elliott RE, Morsi A, Tanweer O, Grobelny B, Geller E, Carlson C, et al. Efficacy of vagus nerve stimulation over time: Review of 65 consecutive patients with treatment-resistant epilepsy treated with VNS >10years. Epilepsy and Behavior. 2011;**20**:478-483. DOI: 10.1016/j.yebeh.2010.12.042

[8] Guo Z, Mo J, Zhang C, Zhang J, Hu W, Zhang K. Brain-clinical signatures for vagus nerve stimulation response. CNS Neuroscience & Therapeutics. Mar 2023;**29**(3):855-865. DOI: 10.1111/cns.14021

[9] Hamilton P, Soryal I, Dhahri P, al. et. Clinical outcomes of VNS therapy with AspireSR((R)) (including cardiac-based seizure detection) at a large complex epilepsy and surgery Centre. Seizure. 2018;**58**:120-126

[10] Verlinden TJM, Rijkers K, Hoogland G, Herrler A. Morphology of the human cervical vagus nerve: Implications for vagus nerve stimulation treatment. Acta Neurologica Scandinavica. 2016;**133**:173-182. DOI: 10.1111/ane.12462

[11] Finger S. Benjamin Franklin, electricity, and the palsies. Neurology. 2006;**66**:1559-1563. DOI: 10.1212/01.WNL.0000216159.60623.2B

[12] Magiorkinis E, Diamantis A, Sidiropoulou K, Panteliadis C. Highights in the history of epilepsy: The last 200 years. Epilepsy Research and Treatment. 2014;**2014**:1-13. DOI: 10.1155/2014/582039

[13] Woodbury DM, Woodbury JW. Effects of vagal stimulation on experimentally induced seizures in rats. Epilepsia. 1990;**31**(Suppl. 2):S7-S19. DOI: 10.1111/J.1528-1157.1990.TB05852.X

[14] Zabara J. Peripheral control of hypersynchronous discharge in epilepsy. Electroencephalography and Clinical Neurophysiology. 1985;**61**:S162. DOI: 10.1016/0013-4694(85)90626-1

[15] Handforth A, DeGiorgio C, Schachter S, al. et. Vagus nerve stimulation therapy for partial-onset seizures: A randomized active-control trial. Neurology. 1998;**51**:48-55

[16] Uthman BM, Reichl AM, Dean JC, Eisenschenk S, Gilmore R, Reid S, et al. Effectiveness of vagus nerve stimulation in epilepsy patients: A 12-year observation. Neurology. 2004;**63**:1124-1126. DOI: 10.1212/01.WNL.0000138499.87068.C0

[17] Sackeim HA, Rush AJ, George MS, Marangell LB, Husain MM, Nahas Z, et al. Vagus nerve stimulation (VNS™) for treatment-resistant depression: Efficacy, side effects, and predictors of outcome. Neuropsychopharmacology. 2001;**25**(5):713-728. DOI: 10.1016/s0893-133x(01)00271-8

[18] Terra VC, Furlanetti LL, Aparecido A, Thomé U, Akico M, Sakamoto AC, et al. Epilepsy & Behavior Vagus nerve stimulation in pediatric patients : Is it really worthwhile ? Epilepsy & Behavior. 2014;**31**:329-333. DOI: 10.1016/j.yebeh.2013.10.011

[19] Elliott RE, Morsi A, Geller EB, Carlson CC, Devinsky O, Doyle WK. Impact of failed intracranial epilepsy surgery on the effectiveness of subsequent vagus nerve stimulation. Neurosurgery. 2011;**69**:1210-1217. DOI: 10.1227/NEU.0b013e3182230ae3

[20] Krahl S, Clark K, Smith D, Browning R. Locus coeruleus lesions suppress the seizure-attenuating effects of vagus nerve stimulation. Epilepsia. 1998;**39**:709-714

[21] Raedt R, Clinckers R, Mollet L, Vonck K, El Tahry R, Wyckhuys T, et al. Increased hippocampal noradrenaline is a biomarker for efficacy of vagus nerve stimulation in a limbic seizure model. Journal of Neurochemistry. 2011;**117**:461-469. DOI: 10.1111/J.1471-4159.2011.07214.X

[22] Berger A, Vespa S, Dricot L, Dumoulin M, Iachim E, Doguet P, et al. How is the norepinephrine system involved in the antiepileptic effects of Vagus nerve stimulation? Frontiers in Neuroscience. 2 Dec 2021;**15**:790943. DOI: 10.3389/fnins.2021.790943

[23] Aston-Jones G, Ennis M, Pieribone VA, Nickell WT, Shipley MT. The brain nucleus locus coeruleus: Restricted afferent control of a broad efferent network. Science (1979). 1986;**234**:734-737. DOI: 10.1126/SCIENCE.3775363

[24] Walker BR, Easton A, Gale K. Regulation of limbic motor seizures by GABA and glutamate transmission in nucleus tractus solitarius. Epilepsia. 1999;**40**:1051-1057. DOI: 10.1111/J.1528-1157.1999.TB00818.X

[25] Sangare A, Marchi A, Pruvost-Robieux E, Soufflet C, Crepon B, Ramdani C, et al. The effectiveness of Vagus nerve stimulation in drug-resistant epilepsy correlates with Vagus nerve stimulation-induced electroencephalography desynchronization. Brain Connectivity. 2020;**10**:566. DOI: 10.1089/BRAIN.2020.0798

[26] Bodin C, Aubert S, Daquin G, Carron R, Scavarda D, McGonigal A, et al. Responders to vagus nerve stimulation (VNS) in refractory epilepsy have reduced interictal cortical synchronicity on scalp EEG. Epilepsy Research. 2015;**113**:98-103. DOI: 10.1016/j.eplepsyres.2015.03.018

[27] Henry TR, Bakay RAE, Votaw JR, Pennell PB, Epstein CM, Faber TL, Grafton ST, Hoffman JM. Brain blood

flow alterations induced by therapeutic vagus nerve stimulation in partial epilepsy: I. acute effects at high and low levels of stimulation. Epilepsia. Sep 1998;**39**(9):983-990. DOI: 10.1111/j.1528-1157.1998.tb01448.x

[28] Henry TR, Votaw JR, Pennell PB, Epstein CM, Bakay RAE, Faber TL, et al. Acute blood flow changes and efficacy of vagus nerve stimulation in partial epilepsy. Neurology. 1999;**52**:1166-1173. DOI: 10.1212/WNL.52.6.1166

[29] Henry TR, Bakay RAE, Pennell PB, Epstein CM, Votaw JR. Brain blood-flow alterations induced by therapeutic vagus nerve stimulation in partial epilepsy: II. Prolonged effects at high and low levels of stimulation. Epilepsia. 2004;**45**:1064-1070. DOI: 10.1111/j.0013-9580.2004.03104.x

[30] Bonaz B, Sinniger V, Pellissier S. The vagus nerve in the neuro-immune axis: Implications in the pathology of the gastrointestinal tract. Frontiers in Immunology. 2 Nov 2017;**8**:1452. DOI: 10.3389/fimmu.2017.01452. PMID: 29163522; PMCID: PMC5673632

[31] Koopman FA, Chavan SS, Miljko S, Grazio S, Sokolovic S, Schuurman PR, et al. Vagus nerve stimulation inhibits cytokine production and attenuates disease severity in rheumatoid arthritis. Proceedings of the National Academy of Sciences of the United States of America. 2016;**113**:8284-8289. DOI: 10.1073/PNAS.1605635113

[32] Alexander GM, Huang YZ, Soderblom EJ, He XP, Moseley MA, McNamara JO. Vagal nerve stimulation modifies neuronal activity and the proteome of excitatory synapses of amygdala/piriform cortex. Journal of Neurochemistry. 2017;**140**:629-644. DOI: 10.1111/JNC.13931

[33] Jain P, Arya R. Vagus nerve stimulation and seizure outcomes in Pediatric refractory epilepsy: Systematic review and Meta-analysis. Neurology. 2021;**96**:1041-1051. DOI: 10.1212/WNL.0000000000012030

[34] Xie H, Ma J, Ji T, Liu Q, Cai L, Wu Y. Efficacy of vagus nerve stimulation in 95 children of drug-resistant epilepsy with structural etiology. Epilepsy and Behavior. Mar 2023;**140**:109107. DOI: 10.1016/j.yebeh.2023.109107. Epub 2023 Feb 7. PMID: 36758359

[35] Kayyali H, Abdelmoity S, Bansal L, Kaufman C, Smith K, Fecske E, et al. The efficacy and safety of rapid cycling Vagus nerve stimulation in children with intractable epilepsy. Pediatric Neurology. 2020;**109**:35-38. DOI: 10.1016/j.pediatrneurol.2020.04.003

[36] Wilfong AA, Schultz RJ. Vagus nerve stimulation for treatment of epilepsy in Rett syndrome. Developmental Medicine and Child Neurology. 2006;**48**:683-686. DOI: 10.1111/J.1469-8749.2006.TB01340.X

[37] Wilfong. Vagus nerve stimulation for treatment of epilepsy in Rett syndrome. Developmental Medicine & Child Neurology. Wiley Online Library. Aug 2006;**48**(8):683-686. DOI: 10.1017/S0012162206001435. PMID: 16836782. Available from: https://onlinelibrary.wiley.com/doi/abs/10.1111/j.1469-8749.2006.tb01340.x?sid=nlm%3Apubmed [Accessed: March 27, 2023]

[38] Tomei KL, Mau CY, Ghali M, Pak J, Goldstein IM. Vagal nerve stimulation for medically refractory epilepsy in Angelman syndrome: A series of three cases. Child's Nervous System. 2018;**34**:395-400. DOI: 10.1007/S00381-018-3723-Z

[39] Youn SE, Jung DE, Kang HC, Kim HD. Long-term results of vagus

nerve stimulation in children with Dravet syndrome: Time-dependent, delayed antiepileptic effect. Epilepsy Research. Aug 2021;**174**:106665. DOI: 10.1016/j.eplepsyres.2021.106665. Epub 2021 May 8. PMID: 34000601

[40] Ding J, Wang L, Li W, Wang Y, Jiang S, Xiao L, et al. Up to what extent does Dravet syndrome benefit from Neurostimulation techniques? Frontiers in Neurology. 13 Apr 2022;**13**:843975. DOI: 10.3389/fneur.2022.843975. PMID: 35493838; PMCID: PMC9044920

[41] Parain D, Penniello MJ, Berquen P, Delangre T, Billard C, Murphy JV. Vagal nerve stimulation in tuberous sclerosis complex patients. Pediatric Neurology. 2001;**25**:213-216. DOI: 10.1016/s0887-8994(01)00312-5

[42] Tong X, Wang X, Qin L, Zhou J, Guan Y, Teng P, et al. Vagus nerve stimulation for drug-resistant epilepsy induced by tuberous sclerosis complex. Epilepsy and Behavior. Jan 2022;**126**:108431. DOI: 10.1016/j.yebeh.2021.108431. Epub 2021 Dec 6. PMID: 34883463

[43] Hadjinicolaou A, Jain P, Arya R, et al. Generator replacement with cardiac-based VNS device in children with drug-resistant epilepsy: An observational study. Epilepsy Research. 2020;**167**:106431. DOI: 10.1016/j.eplepsyres.2020.106431. ISSN 0920-1211

[44] Nagarajan L, Walsh P, Gregory P, Lee M. VNS therapy in clinical practice in children with refractory epilepsy. Acta Neurologica Scandinavica. 2002;**105**:13-17. DOI: 10.1034/J.1600-0404.2002.00129.X

[45] Orosz I, McCormick D, Zamponi N, Varadkar S, Feucht M, Parain D, et al. Vagus nerve stimulation for drug-resistant epilepsy: A European long-term study up to 24 months in 347 children. Epilepsia. 2014;**55**:1576-1584. DOI: 10.1111/EPI.12762

[46] Abdelmoity SA, Abdelmoity AA, Riordan SM, Kaufman C, Le Pichon JB, Abdelmoity A. The efficacy and tolerability of auto-stimulation-VNS in children with Lennox-Gastaut syndrome. Seizure. 2021;**86**:168-174. DOI: 10.1016/J.SEIZURE.2021.02.015

[47] Tsai JD, Chang YC, Lin LC, Hung KL, on behalf of the VNS TCNS. The neuropsychological outcome of pediatric patients with refractory epilepsy treated with VNS - a 24-month follow-up in Taiwan. Epilepsy and Behavior. Mar 2016;**56**:95-98. DOI: 10.1016/j.yebeh.2015.12.030. Epub 2016 Feb 4. PMID: 26851647

[48] Jain P, Arya R. Vagus nerve stimulation and seizure outcomes in Pediatric refractory epilepsy. Neurology. 2021;**96**:1041-1051. DOI: 10.1212/WNL.0000000000012030

[49] Englot DJ, Chang EF, Auguste KI. Vagus nerve stimulation for epilepsy: A meta-analysis of efficacy and predictors of response. Journal of Neurosurgery. 2011;**115**:1248-1255. DOI: 10.3171/2011.7JNS11977

[50] Englot D, Chang E, Auguste K. Efficacy of vagus nerve stimulation for epilepsy by patient age, epilepsy duration, and seizure type. Neurosurgery Clinics of North America. 2011;**22**:443-448

[51] Wheless JW, Gienapp AJ, Ryvlin P. Vagus nerve stimulation (VNS) therapy update. Epilepsy & Behavior. 2018;**88**:2-10

[52] Kawai K, Tanaka T, Baba H, Bunker M, Ikeda A, Inoue Y, et al.

Outcome of vagus nerve stimulation for drug-resistant epilepsy: The first three years of a prospective Japanese registry. Epileptic Disorders. 2017;**19**:327-338. DOI: 10.1684/epd.2017.0929

[53] Englot D, Rolston J, Wright C, Hassnain K, Chang E. Rates and predictors of seizure freedom with vagus nerve stimulation for intractable epilepsy. Neurosurgery. 2016;**79**:345-353

[54] Cramer SC, Sur M, Dobkin BH, O'Brien C, Sanger TD, Trojanowski JQ, et al. Harnessing neuroplasticity for clinical applications. Brain. 2011;**134**:1591-1609. DOI: 10.1093/BRAIN/AWR039

[55] Kim JS, Lee DE, Bae H, Song JY, Yang KI, Hong SB. Effects of Vagus nerve stimulation on sleep-disordered breathing, daytime sleepiness, and sleep quality in patients with drug-resistant epilepsy. Journal of Clinical Neurology. 2022;**18**:315. DOI: 10.3988/jcn.2022.18.3.315

[56] Parhizgar F, Nugent K, Raj R. Obstructive sleep Apnea and respiratory complications associated with Vagus nerve stimulators. Journal of Clinical Sleep Medicine. 2011;**07**:401-407. DOI: 10.5664/JCSM.1204

[57] Sirven JI, Sperling M, Naritoku D, Schachter S, Labar D, Holmes M, et al. Vagus nerve stimulation therapy for epilepsy in older adults. Neurology. 2000;**54**:1179-1182. DOI: 10.1212/WNL.54.5.1179

[58] Vonck K, Raedt R, Naulaerts J, De Vogelaere F, Thiery E, Van Roost D, et al. Vagus nerve stimulation…25 years later! What do we know about the effects on cognition? Neuroscience and Biobehavioral Reviews. 2014;**45**:63-71. DOI: 10.1016/j.neubiorev.2014.05.005

[59] Broncel A, Bocian R, Kłos-Wojtczak P, Kulbat-Warycha K, Konopacki J. Vagal nerve stimulation as a promising tool in the improvement of cognitive disorders. Brain Research Bulletin. 2020;**155**:37-47. DOI: 10.1016/j.brainresbull.2019.11.011

[60] Vargas-Caballero M, Warming H, Walker R, Holmes C, Cruickshank G, Patel B. Vagus nerve stimulation as a potential therapy in early Alzheimer's disease: A review. Frontiers in Human Neuroscience. 29 Apr 2022;**16**:866434. DOI: 10.3389/fnhum.2022.866434. PMID: 35572001; PMCID: PMC9098960

[61] Helmers SL, Begnaud J, Cowley A, Corwin HM, Edwards JC, Holder DL, et al. Application of a computational model of vagus nerve stimulation. Acta Neurologica Scandinavica. 2012;**126**:336-343. DOI: 10.1111/J.1600-0404.2012.01656.X

[62] Fahoum F, Boffini M, Kann L, Faini S, Gordon C, Tzadok M, et al. VNS parameters for clinical response in epilepsy. Brain Stimulation. 2022;**15**:814-821. DOI: 10.1016/J.BRS.2022.05.016

[63] Kulju T, Haapasalo J, Rainesalo S, Lehtimaki K, Peltola J. Autostimulation in vagus nerve stimulator treatment: Modulating neuromodulation. Neuromodulation. 2019;**22**:630-637

[64] Lo WB, Chevill B, Philip S, Agrawal S, Walsh AR. Seizure improvement following vagus nerve stimulator (VNS) battery change with cardiac-based seizure detection automatic stimulation (AutoStim): Early experience in a regional paediatric unit. Child's Nervous System. 2021;**37**:1237-1241. DOI: 10.1007/S00381-020-04962-3

Section 3

Society and Epilepsy

Chapter 7

Perspective Chapter: Stigma and Its Impact on People Living with Epilepsy in Rural Communities

Thendo Gertie Makhado and Lufuno Makhado

Abstract

Epilepsy is a neurological condition affecting millions worldwide, especially in low- and middle-income countries. This condition is poorly understood, and various misconceptions surround it, leading to stigma toward people living with epilepsy (PLWE). In rural areas, cultural beliefs and practices significantly shape attitudes toward health and illness, exacerbating the stigma associated with epilepsy. This proposed book addresses the pervasive stigma experienced by individuals living with epilepsy in rural communities. Through a review of relevant literature and case studies, this chapter examines how stigma affects the lives of people with epilepsy in rural areas. The chapter also explores strategies for reducing stigma, including community-based education and awareness programmes and the role of healthcare providers in promoting understanding and acceptance of epilepsy. In general, this chapter aims to highlight the need for increased awareness and understanding of epilepsy and its impact on those living with the condition in rural communities. It is believed that by tackling the stigma associated with epilepsy and promoting inclusivity, the quality of life of people living with epilepsy may be improved.

Keywords: epilepsy, stigma, rural communities, neurological disorder, misconceptions

1. Introduction

Stigma is the rejection of or prejudice against a person or group based on attributes that are thought to set them apart from other members of society [1, 2]. Therefore, it means that an individual may be rejected or discriminated against because of their skin colour, conditions, culture, and language. Arias-Colmenero et al. [3]; Aubé et al. [4]; Kwon et al. [5] stated that there are different kinds of stigma which include self-stigma, perceived stigma, social stigma, healthcare practitioner stigma, enacted stigma, and felt stigma and these different kinds of stigma lead to social isolation. Epilepsy, a neurological disorder characterised by recurrent seizures, affects millions of individuals worldwide, making it one of the most common neurological conditions globally [6]. Unfortunately, people living with epilepsy (PLWE) often experience stigma and discrimination due to misconceptions and misunderstandings about the condition [7, 8]. Moreover, this neurological condition is estimated to affect about 50 million people worldwide, and despite its prevalence, it remains a highly stigmatised condition in many societies, including rural communities [9, 10]. In rural communities, cultural beliefs, traditions, and superstitions often significantly shape attitudes toward health and illness [11]. Several misconceptions and myths are attached to epilepsy in different settings, especially rural communities [8, 12]. Some of the misconceptions about epilepsy include that epilepsy is a condition from supernatural powers linked with witchcraft [12, 13]. These misconceptions and myths surrounding epilepsy can be deeply ingrained within the fabric of these communities, leading to fear, discrimination, social isolation and stigmatisation of individuals with epilepsy [11, 13, 14]. Moreover, limited awareness of epilepsy in rural communities, poor healthcare, and lack of resources in rural areas intensifies the challenges faced by people living with epilepsy (PLWE) and it hinders their ability to address and combat stigma [15, 16].

Understanding the impact of stigma on PLWE in rural communities is crucial for developing targeted interventions and support systems. Addressing the underlying factors contributing to stigma, such as cultural beliefs and misconceptions, can promote greater awareness, acceptance, and inclusivity within these communities [17]. Enhancing knowledge about epilepsy, its causes, and its management can help dispel myths and reduce the fear associated with the condition [15, 18].

1.1 Background

This chapter focuses on the influence of stigma on people living with epilepsy in rural areas. Epilepsy is a neurological condition that causes repeated seizures and affects millions worldwide [19–21]. Despite its frequency and impact on people's lives, PLWE is commonly stigmatised and discriminated against due to widespread misconceptions and misunderstandings about the disorder. These social barriers can exacerbate the challenges that people with epilepsy face and hinder their ability to participate fully in society.

Stigma is a social phenomenon characterised by negative attitudes, beliefs, and stereotypes, marginalising and excluding individuals with certain health conditions [22–25]. In the case of epilepsy, stigma arises from a combination of cultural beliefs, superstitions, and a lack of understanding about the nature of the disorder. This stigma is especially prevalent in rural communities, where cultural beliefs and practices considerably influence attitudes about health and illness [5, 26–29]. In many rural areas, cultural beliefs attribute epilepsy to supernatural causes, such as possession or divine punishment [30–33]. These beliefs stigmatise people with epilepsy, causing fear, prejudice, and social exclusion [5, 34–36]. Furthermore, poor access to healthcare, education, and resources in rural regions exacerbates the difficulties faced by people with epilepsy, making it difficult for them to address and battle stigma [5, 34, 37, 38].

This chapter aims to provide an educational analysis of the influence of stigma on people living with epilepsy in rural settings. The chapter highlights the problems individuals with epilepsy confront in obtaining healthcare, jobs, and education in rural locations by evaluating relevant literature and case studies. It also investigates the psychological and social effects of stigma on the well-being of people with epilepsy. The chapter also looks into initiatives for stigma reduction, including community-based education and awareness campaigns, as well as the role of healthcare personnel in increasing epilepsy understanding and acceptance. These efforts aim to reduce stigma, enhance healthcare and support systems access, and encourage inclusion in rural communities. Overall, the academic foundation of this chapter is based on scholarly research on epilepsy, stigma, and the unique obstacles that people with epilepsy encounter in rural settings. The chapter intends to provide a comprehensive overview of the subject by evaluating existing literature and drawing on empirical evidence, emphasising the need for better awareness, assistance, and inclusion for those with epilepsy in rural settings.

1.2 Purpose of the chapter

This chapter aims to shed light on the adverse effects of stigma on people living with epilepsy who live in rural regions and provide a complete understanding of their difficulties. It aims to increase awareness of the unique dynamics of epilepsy-related stigma in rural communities, where cultural attitudes and insufficient access to resources are significant considerations. The chapter emphasises the urgent need to address these concerns by evaluating the influence of stigma on numerous elements of persons' lives, such as healthcare access, employment, education, and social well-being. The chapter also looks at techniques and interventions that might help eliminate stigma and increase inclusivity, such as community-based education initiatives and the involvement of healthcare providers. The overarching goal is to promote improved awareness, acceptance, and support for those living with epilepsy in rural settings. This ensures that people have equal access to resources and opportunities for leading whole lives free of stigma and discrimination.

2. Stigma and its impact

2.1 Stigma and misconceptions about epilepsy

The stigma surrounding epilepsy arises from misconceptions, stereotypes, and cultural beliefs that contribute to the social marginalisation and discrimination experienced by individuals with the condition [9, 34, 36]. Epilepsy is typically buried in misconceptions and misunderstandings in many communities, particularly rural ones, exacerbating its associated stigma. The belief that epilepsy is communicable is a prevalent misconception. This idea derives from a misunderstanding of the disorder's neurological origins. People may mistakenly fear that they can contract epilepsy through close contact with individuals with seizures, leading to social distancing and isolation of those with the condition [34, 36, 39]. Such views not only contribute to the stigmatisation of people with epilepsy but also impede their social interactions and integration into their communities.

Another common misconception is that epilepsy is a mental illness or a form of insanity [9, 40–42]. This perception arises due to seizures' visible and sometimes unpredictable nature, which can be misinterpreted as signs of insanity. PLWE often face negative labels and are unjustly associated with cognitive impairments or psychological instability. These false assumptions reinforce stigma and affect individuals' self-esteem and self-perception [34].

Cultural beliefs and superstitions significantly influence the perception of epilepsy in many rural communities [8, 34, 37, 43, 44]. Some cultures attribute seizures to spiritual or supernatural causes, associating them with curses, evil spirits, or divine punishment. This attribution of mystical causes to epilepsy further stigmatises affected individuals, leading to social exclusion, fear, and discrimination [45, 46]. Such cultural beliefs can contribute to people's unwillingness to seek medical care, instead turning to traditional healers or participating in dangerous acts to eliminate imagined supernatural forces [47–49].

Challenging these assumptions and cultural ideas is critical to eliminate epilepsy-related stigma. Public education efforts, community discussions, and sharing of culturally relevant information can help debunk myths and improve knowledge of epilepsy as a neurological disorder. It is possible to demystify epilepsy and build a more inclusive and supportive environment for PLWE in rural communities by encouraging an accurate understanding of its causes, triggers, and management.

2.2 Challenges in healthcare access

Access to healthcare services is fundamental to managing epilepsy and mitigating its impact on individuals' lives. However, in rural communities, people with epilepsy face numerous challenges that hinder their ability to access appropriate healthcare, exacerbating the burden of the condition.

One primary challenge is the limited availability and accessibility of healthcare facilities in rural areas [15, 50, 51]. These communities often suffer from inadequate healthcare infrastructure, including a scarcity of hospitals, clinics, and specialised epilepsy centres [16, 37, 52]. Consequently, individuals affected by epilepsy might be compelled to undertake extensive journeys to access necessary medical care, leading to physical and financial hardships, especially for those with limited means. The stigma surrounding epilepsy adds another layer of complexity to healthcare access. Many individuals with epilepsy in rural communities fear the negative judgements and discrimination they might face when seeking medical care [9, 34]. As a result, individuals may postpone or avoid obtaining treatment entirely, resulting in suboptimal management of their condition and an increased risk of consequences. Similarly, it was revealed that one of the contributing factors to poor health-seeking behaviour for PLWE is due to stigma and fear of being recognised as a person living with epilepsy, which can lead to discrimination and social isolation [50].

Healthcare providers in rural areas may also lack the necessary knowledge and training to diagnose and treat epilepsy effectively. This gap in lacking knowledge related to epilepsy results in misdiagnosis or underdiagnosis of patients, which further delays appropriate care [53]. Moreover, the scarcity of epilepsy specialists and neurologists in rural areas means that individuals may not have access to specialised care or comprehensive treatment plans [54].

Financial constraints pose yet another barrier to healthcare access for individuals with epilepsy in rural communities. Many rural populations face poverty and limited financial resources, making it challenging to afford transportation costs, diagnostic tests, medications, and ongoing medical expenses associated with managing epilepsy [15]. This financial burden can significantly impact their ability to seek and receive adequate healthcare services.

Addressing these challenges requires multifaceted approaches. Improving healthcare infrastructure in rural areas, including the establishment of epilepsy clinics and the deployment of trained healthcare professionals, can enhance access to quality care [55]. Additionally, community-based awareness programmes can educate individuals about epilepsy, dispel myths and misconceptions, and reduce stigma, encouraging affected individuals to seek medical attention without fear of discrimination [56].

The awareness may also be extended by teaching epilepsy from a tender age in schools [18]. Collaborations between healthcare providers, community organisations, and policymakers are vital in implementing these strategies and ensuring that individuals with epilepsy in rural communities receive the care they need.

2.3 Employment and education

The stigma associated with epilepsy in rural communities has significant implications for the employment and educational opportunities available to individuals with the condition [57]. Discrimination and prejudice often create barriers that hinder their ability to secure and maintain employment and access quality education.

In employment, individuals with epilepsy often face discrimination due to misconceptions and unfounded fears about their condition. Employers may harbour concerns about potential safety risks if individuals with epilepsy cannot perform their work-related duties effectively or pose a liability in the workplace [58, 59]. This stigma can result in limited job prospects, lower wages, and a lack of career advancement opportunities for individuals with epilepsy in rural communities [60]. Consequently, affected individuals may experience financial difficulties and dependency on social support systems, further perpetuating the cycle of stigma and exclusion.

Moreover, the fear of revealing their epilepsy diagnosis to employers can lead to secrecy and non-disclosure, as individuals attempt to avoid potential discrimination [34]. This fear stems from the stigma associated with epilepsy and the anticipation of adverse reactions from employers and colleagues. Such concealment may exacerbate workplace stress and anxiety, potentially compromising job performance, and overall well-being.

In the realm of education, individuals with epilepsy in rural communities may encounter obstacles that impede their access to quality education. Stigma and misconceptions about epilepsy can lead to exclusion from educational opportunities or limited support within educational institutions [61]. Teachers, administrators, and peers may lack awareness and understanding of epilepsy, resulting in a lack of appropriate accommodations and support for affected students [8]. Consequently, individuals with epilepsy may experience academic difficulties, reduced educational attainment, and diminished prospects for future employment.

Addressing these challenges requires concerted efforts to promote inclusivity and combat stigma in employment and educational settings. Awareness campaigns and education programmes targeted at employers can help dispel misconceptions about epilepsy, emphasise the abilities and rights of individuals with epilepsy, and foster inclusive workplace environments [62, 63]. Implementing reasonable accommodations, such as flexible work schedules or modifications in job tasks, can support the needs of individuals with epilepsy without compromising workplace safety [63].

In the education sector, promoting epilepsy awareness among educators, students, and parents is crucial. Training programmes can equip educators with the knowledge and skills to provide appropriate support, accommodations, and an inclusive learning environment for students with epilepsy [62]. Additionally, fostering peer education and understanding can help reduce bullying, promote empathy, and create a supportive atmosphere for students with epilepsy.

By addressing employment and educational barriers through proactive measures and promoting inclusive practices, rural communities can ensure that individuals with epilepsy have equal opportunities for employment, career advancement, and educational success.

2.4 Social and psychological well-being

The stigma surrounding epilepsy in rural communities profoundly impacts the social and psychological well-being of individuals living with the condition [34, 64]. Stigmatisation often leads to social exclusion, isolation, and strained relationships, causing significant emotional and psychological distress.

One of the main consequences of epilepsy-related stigma is the sense of isolation experienced by individuals with the condition. Stigma can create barriers to social interactions, as people may fear associating with someone with epilepsy due to misunderstandings and fears about seizures [34, 64]. This social isolation can lead to feelings of loneliness, low self-esteem, and a diminished sense of belonging within their communities.

Stigma also affects personal relationships and may strain familial and friendship ties. Families and friends may experience internalised stigma, where the affected individual and their family members internalise negative beliefs and feelings about epilepsy [34, 65]. This can lead to strained relationships, secrecy, and a lack of open communication about the condition within the family unit. Friends and acquaintances may distance themselves from individuals with epilepsy due to fear, lack of understanding, or discomfort, further contributing to feelings of social exclusion and alienation.

The psychological impact of epilepsy-related stigma can be significant. Individuals with epilepsy often experience heightened anxiety, depression, and diminished self-worth because of the negative societal attitudes they encounter [61]. Fear of public judgement and discrimination can lead to increased stress levels, social anxiety, and avoidance of social situations. This psychological burden can have detrimental effects on overall well-being, quality of life, and the ability to engage in meaningful activities.

In rural communities where access to mental health support may be limited, individuals with epilepsy may face additional challenges in accessing appropriate psychological care [16]. The lack of mental health resources compounds the already existing barriers to social and psychological well-being, further underscoring the need for comprehensive support systems [16].

Community-based support programmes and advocacy initiatives are crucial to address the social and psychological challenges associated with epilepsy-related stigma [62]. Support groups, both in-person and online, can provide individuals with epilepsy with a sense of belonging, opportunities for peer support, and a safe space to share their experiences [66]. These groups can help individuals develop coping strategies, build resilience, and normalise their experiences.

Education and awareness campaigns to challenge stigmatise beliefs and promote understanding within communities are also essential [7, 61]. By increasing knowledge about epilepsy, its causes, and its management, communities can foster empathy, reduce fear, and promote inclusivity [62]. Cultivating an environment that encourages open dialogue, acceptance, and support can help alleviate the social and psychological burdens of individuals with epilepsy in rural communities.

3. Strategies for reducing stigma

Reducing the stigma associated with epilepsy in rural communities requires a multifaceted approach that involves education, awareness, and community engagement. Implementing strategies to combat stigma can foster understanding, empathy, and acceptance, creating more inclusive environments for individuals with epilepsy.

Community-Based Education and Awareness Programmes: Community-based education programmes play a vital role in dispelling myths, challenging misconceptions, and promoting accurate knowledge about epilepsy. These programmes can be conducted through workshops, public forums, and interactive sessions, engaging community members, healthcare providers, educators, and religious leaders [7]. This can also be done by educating learners from the primary level so that when they grow up, they are knowledgeable about the condition, which may decrease stigma related to epilepsy [62]. By addressing cultural beliefs, superstitions, and misunderstandings, these initiatives can help reshape attitudes and reduce the stigma surrounding epilepsy.

Advocacy and Support Groups: Establishing advocacy and support groups specifically focused on epilepsy can provide a platform for individuals with epilepsy, their families, and allies to come together, share experiences, and raise awareness [66]. These groups can engage in advocacy efforts to promote policies that protect the rights of individuals with epilepsy and combat discrimination. They can also serve as sources of emotional support, empowerment, and education, helping individuals navigate the challenges associated with living with epilepsy in rural communities.

Promoting Role Models and Personal Narratives: Highlighting positive stories and personal narratives of individuals with epilepsy can challenge stereotypes and humanise the condition [66]. Sharing stories of resilience, achievements, and successful management of epilepsy can inspire others and contribute to de-stigmatisation efforts. Role models who have excelled in various fields despite living with epilepsy can serve as powerful examples, showcasing the abilities and potential of individuals with epilepsy.

Collaboration with Healthcare Providers: Healthcare providers are crucial in reducing stigma and promoting understanding of epilepsy [67]. Through training programmes and continuous medical education, healthcare professionals can develop the knowledge and skills necessary to provide appropriate care, support, and guidance to individuals with epilepsy [68]. They can also play a vital role in educating the broader community about epilepsy, dispelling myths, and promoting inclusive attitudes.

Promoting Inclusive Policies and Legislation: Governments and policymakers are responsible for enacting and enforcing inclusive policies that protect the rights of individuals with epilepsy and prevent discrimination. These policies can encompass employment protections, anti-stigma campaigns, educational accommodations, and access to healthcare services [62, 69, 70]. By promoting legislation that addresses stigma and discrimination, rural communities can create an environment that fosters inclusivity, equal opportunities, and social integration for individuals with epilepsy.

Evaluation and Continuous Improvement: It is essential to evaluate the effectiveness of stigma reduction strategies and make necessary adjustments based on feedback and outcomes. Regular assessments can help identify gaps, measure the impact of interventions, and refine strategies for maximum effectiveness [71]. By implementing these strategies, rural communities can actively work toward reducing stigma, promoting acceptance, and creating a supportive environment that enables individuals with epilepsy to live fulfilling lives without fear of judgement or exclusion.

Promoting Inclusivity in Rural Communities: Promoting inclusivity in rural communities is essential to create an environment that embraces individuals with epilepsy and ensures their equal participation, rights, and opportunities [72]. By addressing stigma and fostering understanding and acceptance, rural communities can work toward building a supportive and inclusive society for individuals with epilepsy.

Community Education and Sensitisation: Community-wide education and sensitisation initiatives are crucial in promoting inclusivity. These programmes can be designed to raise awareness about epilepsy, challenge misconceptions, and foster empathy and understanding. Workshops, public forums, and information campaigns can engage community members, schools, religious institutions, and local organisations, helping to dispel stigma and build a foundation of knowledge and acceptance [8, 62].

Accessible Healthcare Services: Enhancing access to healthcare services is vital for individuals with epilepsy in rural areas. Establishing epilepsy clinics, mobile health units, and telemedicine services can help bridge the gap in healthcare access. Collaborations between healthcare providers, community organisations, and government agencies can ensure that quality epilepsy care is available and affordable. Providing specialised training for healthcare professionals in rural areas can also improve diagnosis, treatment, and support for individuals with epilepsy [73].

Inclusive Policies and Legislation: Rural communities should adopt inclusive policies and legislation that protect the rights and promote the well-being of individuals with epilepsy [74]. These policies include employment protections, educational accommodations, accessibility requirements, and anti-discrimination measures. By aligning with national and international standards, rural communities can ensure that individuals with epilepsy have equal opportunities, fair treatment, and legal safeguards against discrimination.

Support Networks and Peer Mentoring: Establishing support networks and peer mentoring programmes can provide crucial emotional support, guidance, and a sense of belonging to individuals with epilepsy [66]. These networks can be created through local organisations, support groups, or online platforms. Peer mentors who have personal experiences with epilepsy can offer practical advice, encouragement, and understanding, helping individuals navigate the challenges associated with living with epilepsy in rural communities.

Education and Empowerment: Educational institutions play a pivotal role in promoting inclusivity. Schools should provide a safe and supportive environment for students with epilepsy, ensuring that they receive appropriate accommodations and support services. Teachers and school staff can undergo training to enhance their understanding of epilepsy and develop strategies to create an inclusive learning environment. Empowering individuals with epilepsy through education and skills training can enhance their self-esteem, independence, and economic opportunities [8, 18, 62].

Collaborative Partnerships: Promoting inclusivity requires collaboration among various stakeholders, including healthcare providers, educators, community leaders, and individuals with epilepsy and their families. By working together, these stakeholders can share resources, expertise, and ideas to develop comprehensive strategies for inclusivity [62, 69]. Collaborative partnerships can also facilitate the coordination of services, advocacy efforts, and the implementation of initiatives that address the unique needs and challenges faced by individuals with epilepsy in rural communities.

By implementing these strategies, rural communities can promote inclusivity and create an environment where individuals with epilepsy feel valued, supported, and included. By reducing stigma, increasing awareness, and providing necessary resources and support systems, rural communities can empower individuals with epilepsy to lead fulfilling lives and contribute to their communities.

4. Conclusion and future directions

The impact of stigma on individuals living with epilepsy in rural communities is significant and multifaceted. Stigmatisation arises from misconceptions, cultural beliefs, and a lack of understanding about epilepsy. This stigma creates barriers to healthcare access, employment, education, and social inclusion, adversely affecting the social and psychological well-being of individuals with epilepsy. To address these challenges, various strategies can be implemented. Community-based education and awareness programmes can dispel myths, challenge misconceptions, and foster empathy and acceptance. Advocacy and support groups can provide a platform for individuals with epilepsy to share experiences and promote their rights. Collaboration with healthcare providers, inclusive policies and legislation, and promoting support networks and peer mentoring further reduce stigma and promote inclusivity.

Looking to the future, it is essential to continue advancing efforts to combat epilepsy-related stigma in rural communities. This includes ongoing research to understand the cultural and social dynamics contributing to stigma in different contexts. Additionally, evaluating the effectiveness of stigma reduction strategies and refining approaches based on feedback and outcomes is crucial for continuous improvement.

Education and awareness should remain central in future initiatives, targeting the general public and healthcare professionals, educators, and policymakers. By integrating epilepsy education into school curricula, healthcare training programmes, and community outreach initiatives, accurate knowledge about epilepsy can be disseminated more widely, contributing to a more informed and accepting society. Moreover, the development of accessible and affordable healthcare services specifically tailored to the needs of rural communities is essential. This includes increasing the availability of epilepsy clinics, improving access to specialised care, and expanding telemedicine services to reach individuals in remote areas. Additionally, fostering collaboration between healthcare providers, community organisations, and government agencies can strengthen the support network available to individuals with epilepsy.

It is also essential to prioritise empowering individuals with epilepsy through education, skills training, and economic opportunities. By equipping them with the tools and resources necessary for self-advocacy and independence, individuals with epilepsy can actively contribute to their communities and challenge the barriers imposed by stigma. Through efforts to address stigma, promote inclusivity, and provide comprehensive support systems, rural communities can ensure that individuals with epilepsy have equal opportunities, access to healthcare, and a supportive environment that enables them to lead fulfilling lives. Through continued efforts, research, and collaboration, we can strive for a future where epilepsy-related stigma is minimised, and individuals with epilepsy are embraced as valued members of their communities.

5. Summary of the chapter

This chapter focused on the complex stigma surrounding epilepsy in rural communities and its far-reaching effects on various aspects of life. The main goal is to shed light on the harmful consequences of this stigma on people living with epilepsy (PLWE) and to raise awareness about the intricate dynamics of epilepsy-related stigma in rural areas. Stigma arises from misunderstandings, stereotypes, and cultural beliefs, leading to the social marginalisation of PLWE. Misconceptions include the false notion that epilepsy is contagious or a sign of insanity. Cultural superstitions link it to curses or divine punishment, further fuelling the stigma. Such misconceptions hinder social integration and can even affect a person's willingness to seek medical care for their condition. In rural communities, accessing proper healthcare infrastructure is already challenging, and stigma adds another layer of complexity. The absence of epilepsy specialists, financial constraints, and fears of discrimination can delay or prevent treatment, resulting in poor management of the condition. To address this, the solutions proposed involve improving healthcare infrastructure, conducting awareness programmes, and promoting collaboration between healthcare providers and community organisations.

The impact of stigma is also evident in employment and education. Discrimination in the workplace due to misconceptions about epilepsy can limit job prospects and career advancement. In the educational sphere, stigma leads to exclusion or inadequate support, which affects academic success. The suggested remedies include education programmes for employers and teachers and implementing reasonable accommodations to support PLWE. Epilepsy-related stigma profoundly affects individuals' social and psychological well-being, leading to isolation, strained familial ties, anxiety, depression, and diminished self-worth. The chapter advocates for community-based support programmes and education campaigns to foster empathy and inclusivity, thus easing the burdens PLWE face in rural areas.

The chapter further provided strategies for reducing the stigma associated with epilepsy in rural communities, including community-based education and awareness programmes to dispel myths, advocacy and support groups, promoting positive role models and personal narratives, collaboration with healthcare providers, promoting inclusive policies and legislation, and continuous evaluation and improvement of interventions. To promote inclusivity in rural communities, initiatives involve community education and sensitisation, accessible healthcare services, inclusive policies and legislation, support networks and peer mentoring, education and empowerment, and collaborative partnerships. By implementing these strategies, rural communities can create a supportive and inclusive environment that empowers individuals with epilepsy to lead fulfilling lives without fear of judgement or exclusion.

Conflict of interest

The authors declare no conflict of interest.

Author details

Thendo Gertie Makhado* and Lufuno Makhado
University of Venda, Thohoyandou, South Africa

*Address all correspondence to: gertie.makhado@univen.ac.za

References

[1] van Veelen R, Veldman J, Van Laar C, Derks B. Distancing from a stigmatized social identity: State of the art and future research agenda on self-group distancing. European Journal of Social Psychology. 2020;**50**(6):1089-1107

[2] Imran N, Afzal H, Aamer I, Hashmi A, Shabbir B, Asif A, et al. Scarlett letter: A study based on experience of stigma by COVID-19 patients in quarantine. Pakistan Journal of Medical Sciences. 2020;**36**(7):1471

[3] Arias-Colmenero T, Pérez-Morente MÁ, Ramos-Morcillo AJ, Capilla-Díaz C, Ruzafa-Martínez M, Hueso-Montoro C. Experiences and attitudes of people with HIV/AIDS: A systematic review of qualitative studies. International Journal of Environmental Research and Public Health. 2020;**17**(2):639

[4] Aubé B, Follenfant A, Goudeau S, Derguy C. Public stigma of autism spectrum disorder at school: Implicit attitudes matter. Journal of Autism and Developmental Disorders. 2021;**51**:1584-1597

[5] Kwon CS, Jacoby A, Ali A, Austin J, Birbeck GL, Braga P, et al. Systematic review of frequency of felt and enacted stigma in epilepsy and determining factors and attitudes toward persons living with epilepsy—Report from the international league against epilepsy task force on stigma in epilepsy. Epilepsia. 2022;**63**(3):573-597

[6] Thijs RD, Surges R, O'Brien TJ, Sander JW. Epilepsy in adults. Lancet. 2019;**393**:689-701

[7] Musekwa OP, Makhado L, Maphula A, Mabunda JT. How much do we know? Assessing public knowledge, awareness, impact, and awareness guidelines for epilepsy: A systematic review. The Open Public Health Journal. 2020;**13**(1)

[8] Makhado TG, Lebese RT, Maputle MS, Makhado L. Epilepsy life skill education guidelines for primary school teachers and learners in Limpopo and Mpumalanga provinces, South Africa: Multiphase mixed methods protocol. PLoS One. 2022;**17**(7):e0271805

[9] Braga P, Hosny H, Kakooza-Mwesige A, Rider F, Tripathi M, Guekht A. How to understand and address the cultural aspects and consequences of diagnosis of epilepsy, including stigma. Epileptic Disorders. 2020;**22**(5):531-547

[10] Anene-Okeke CG, Anosike C, Aluh DO, Odo LE. Secondary school students' knowledge, attitude, and practices towards epilepsy in Nsukka City, Enugu State. Epilepsy & Behavior. 2020;**112**:107441

[11] Mbuba CK, Ngugi AK, Newton CR, Carter JA. The epilepsy treatment gap in developing countries: A systematic review of the magnitude, causes, and intervention strategies. Epilepsia. 2008;**49**(9):1491-1503

[12] Herrmann LK, Welter E, Berg AT, Perzynski AT, Van Doren JR, Sajatovic M. Epilepsy misconceptions and stigma reduction: Current status in Western countries. Epilepsy & Behavior. 2016;**60**:165-173

[13] Kaddumukasa M, Kaddumukasa MN, Buwembo W, Munabi IG, Blixen C, Lhatoo S, et al. Epilepsy misconceptions and stigma reduction interventions in sub-Saharan Africa, a systematic review. Epilepsy & Behavior. 2018;**85**:21-27

[14] Makasi CE, Kilale AM, Ngowi BJ, Lema Y, Katiti V, Mahande MJ, et al. Knowledge and misconceptions about epilepsy among people with epilepsy and their caregivers attending mental health clinics: A qualitative study in Taenia solium endemic pig-keeping communities in Tanzania. Epilepsia Open. 2023;**8**(2):487-496

[15] Kaddumukasa M, Nalubwama H, Kaddumukasa MN, Lhatoo S, Sewankambo N, Katabira E, et al. Barriers to epilepsy care in Central Uganda, a qualitative interview and focus group study involving PLWE and their caregivers. BMC Neurology. 2019;**19**(1):1-10

[16] Lavin B, Dormond C, Scantlebury MH, Frouin PY, Brodie MJ. Bridging the healthcare gap: Building the case for epilepsy virtual clinics in the current healthcare environment. Epilepsy & Behavior. 2020;**111**:107262

[17] Price P, Kobau R, Buelow J, Austin J, Lowenberg K. Improving understanding, promoting social inclusion, and fostering empowerment related to epilepsy: Epilepsy Foundation public awareness campaigns—2001 through 2013. Epilepsy & Behavior. 2015;**44**:239-244

[18] Makhado TG, Lebese RT, Maputle MS. Incorporation of epilepsy into life skills education: Perceptions of primary school learners in Mpumalanga and Limpopo Province—A qualitative exploratory study. Children. 2023;**10**(3):569

[19] Vetri L, Roccella M, Parisi L, Smirni D, Costanza C, Carotenuto M, et al. Epilepsy: A multifaced Spectrum disorder. Behavioral Sciences. 2023;**13**(2):97

[20] Rohira V, Chaudhary S, Das S, Prasad MK. Automatic epilepsy detection from EEG signals. In: Proceedings of the 6th Joint International Conference on Data Science & Management of Data (10th ACM IKDD CODS and 28th COMAD). 2023. pp. 272-273

[21] Liu J, Zhang P, Zou Q, Liang J, Chen Y, Cai Y, et al. Status of epilepsy in the tropics: An overlooked perspective. Epilepsia Open. 2023;**8**(1):32-45

[22] Baierl-Kwok C, Rostosky SS. When worlds collide: The romantic relationship experiences of bisexual-identifying Asian American men. Personal Relationships. 2023. DOI: 10.1111/pere.12496

[23] Granjon M, Odile R, Popa-Roch M, Aubé B, Sanrey C. Breaking the Mold: Disability Stereotyping Is Shaped by Stigma Characteristics. PsyArXiv. 2023. Available from: https://osf.io/43yjc/?view_only=66665a8c73c446e099756ee5cf4fda24

[24] Murvartian L, Saavedra-Macías FJ, de la Mata ML. Public stigmatization of women victims of intimate partner violence by professionals working in the judicial system and law enforcement agencies in Spain. Journal of Interpersonal Violence. 2023;**38**(18-19):08862605231176798

[25] Westbury S, Oyebode O, Van Rens T, Barber TM. Obesity stigma: Causes, consequences, and potential solutions. Current Obesity Reports. 2023;**12**(1):10-23

[26] Kakooza-Mwesige A, Kaddumukasa M, Koltai DC, Kaddumukasa MN, Nakasujja N, Kajumba M, et al. Leveraging the lessons learned from studies on the cultural context of epilepsy care in Uganda: Opportunities and future directions. Epilepsy & Behavior. 2021;**114**:107302

[27] Koltai DC, Smith CE, Cai GY, Ratliff O, Kakooza-Mwesige A, Najjuma JN, et al. Healthcare provider perspectives regarding epilepsy care in Uganda. Epilepsy & Behavior. 2021;**114**:107294

[28] Thapa S, Aro AR. 'Menstruation means impurity': Multilevel interventions are needed to break the menstrual taboo in Nepal. BMC Women's Health. 2021;**21**(1):1-5

[29] Subu MA, Wati DF, Netrida N, Priscilla V, Dias JM, Abraham MS, et al. Types of stigma experienced by patients with mental illness and mental health nurses in Indonesia: A qualitative content analysis. International Journal of Mental Health Systems. 2021;**15**:1-2

[30] Antimov P, Tournev I, Zhelyazkova S, Sander JW. Traditional practices and perceptions of epilepsy among people in Roma communities in Bulgaria. Epilepsy & Behavior. 2020;**108**:107086

[31] Smith CE, Kajumba M, Bobholz S, Smith PJ, Kaddumukasa M, Kakooza-Mwesige A, et al. Pluralistic and singular causal attributions for epilepsy in Uganda. Epilepsy & Behavior. 2021;**114**:107334

[32] Bone I, Dein S. Religion, spirituality, and epilepsy. Epilepsy & Behavior. 2021;**122**:108219

[33] Tayeb HO. Epilepsy stigma in Saudi Arabia: The roles of mind–body dualism, supernatural beliefs, and religiosity. Epilepsy & Behavior. 2019;**95**:175-180

[34] Mayor R, Gunn S, Reuber M, Simpson J. Experiences of stigma in people with epilepsy: A meta-synthesis of qualitative evidence. Seizure. 2022;**94**:142-160

[35] Dayapoglu N, Ayyıldız Nİ, Şeker D. Fear of negative evaluation and the concealment of their disease by epilepsy patients. Epilepsy & Behavior. 2020;**113**:107539

[36] Ali Arazeem A, Tahirah Adedolapo I, Joseph AO. Shame, stigma, and social exclusion: The lived experiences of epileptic patients in a health facility in Ilorin, Nigeria. Global Public Health. 2022;**17**(12):3839-3852

[37] Kissani N, Lengané YT, Patterson V, Mesraoua B, Dawn E, Ozkara C, et al. Telemedicine in epilepsy: How can we improve care, teaching, and awareness? Epilepsy & Behavior. 2020;**103**:106854

[38] Gosain K, Samanta T. Understanding the role of stigma and misconceptions in the experience of epilepsy in India: Findings from a mixed-methods study. Frontiers in Sociology. 13 May 2022;7:790145

[39] Mula M, Kaufman KR. Double stigma in mental health: Epilepsy and mental illness. BJPsych Open. 2020;**6**(4):e72

[40] Abukanna AM, Alenazi MS, Alenazi NS, Alenezi MM, Alanazi IA. Knowledge, attitude and practices of Saudi population in Arar regarding epilepsy and seizures. Medical Science. 2021;**25**(116):2718-2727

[41] Hakami T, Mahfouz M, Najmi H, Adawi A, Hakami R, Areeshi N, et al. Knowledge of and attitude towards epilepsy among university students in Arabia: Misconceptions of the next generation. Epilepsy & Behavior Reports. 2021;**16**:100450

[42] Alsohibani A, Alkheder R, Alharbi M, Alrasheedi M, Alsoghair M, Alsuhaibani M. Public awareness, knowledge, and attitudes

regarding epilepsy in the Qassim region, Saudi Arabia. Epilepsy & Behavior. 2019;**92**:260-264

[43] Chabangu Q, Maputle MS, Lebese RT, Makhado L. Indigenous practices for management of epilepsy by traditional healers in South Africa. Epilepsy and Paroxysmal Conditions. 2022;**14**(3):267-275

[44] Mbelesso P, Luna J, Yangatimbi E, Mboukou C, Preux PM. Sociocultural representations of epilepsy in the Central African Republic: A door-to-door survey. Seizure. 2019;**67**:23-26

[45] Ruesch N. The Stigma of Mental Illness-E-Book: Strategies against Discrimination and Social Exclusion. Chicago, USA: Elsevier Health Sciences; 2022

[46] Koschorke M, Al-Haboubi YH, Tseng PC, Semrau M, Eaton J. Mental health, stigma, and neglected tropical diseases: A review and systematic mapping of the evidence. Frontiers in Tropical Diseases. 2022;**3**:93

[47] Shange S, Ross E. "The question is not how but why things happen": South African traditional healers' explanatory model of mental illness, its diagnosis and treatment. Journal of Cross-Cultural Psychology. 2022;**53**(5):503-521

[48] Kasa GA, Kaba M. Preferences for health care and its determinants among mentally ill patients of the west Shoa zone community, Oromia, Ethiopia. Patient Preference and Adherence. 2023;**17**:557-570

[49] Bademosi F. Cultural and Religious/Spiritual Beliefs and People of African Descent's Attitudes towards Seeking Mental Health Treatment (Doctoral Dissertation, the Chicago School of Professional Psychology). ProQuest LLC. 2020 this is the dessertation from The Chicago School of Professional Psychologys

[50] Molla A, Mekuriaw B, Habtamu E, Mareg M. Treatment-seeking behavior towards epilepsy among rural residents in Ethiopia: A cross-sectional study. Neuropsychiatric Disease and Treatment. 2020;**16**:433-439

[51] Owens S, Sirven JI, Shafer PO, Fishman J, Wild I, Findley M, et al. Innovative approaches reaching underserved and rural communities to improve epilepsy care: A review of the methodology of the connectors project. Epilepsy & Behavior. 2019;**90**:273-283

[52] Kissani N, Cherkaoui Rhazouani O, Souirti Z, Khramaz M, Meryem C, Mebrouk Y, et al. Epilepsy in Morocco: Realities, pitfalls and prospects. Epilepsia Open. 2021;**6**(1):13-21

[53] Mustafa MN, Wedaa Alla LG, Ahmad TK. Knowledge and attitude toward epilepsy among the final and semi-final years medical students at University of Bahri. Sudan. Epilepsia Open. 2022;7(1):144-150

[54] Chin JH. Epilepsy treatment in sub-Saharan Africa: Closing the gap. African Health Sciences. 2012;**12**(2):186-192

[55] Caraballo R, Fejerman N. Management of epilepsy in resource-limited settings. Epileptic Disorders. 2015;**17**(1):13-18

[56] Giuliano L, Cicero CE, Padilla S, Mayaregua DR, Villarreal WM, Sofia V, et al. Knowledge, stigma, and quality of life in epilepsy: Results before and after a community-based epilepsy awareness program in rural Bolivia. Epilepsy & Behavior. 2019;**92**:90-97

[57] Boling W, Means M, Fletcher A. Quality of life and stigma in epilepsy, perspectives from selected regions of Asia and sub-Saharan Africa. Brain Sciences. 2018;**8**(4):59

[58] Day E. Time to end the stigma of epilepsy. Lancet Neurology. 2022;**21**:671

[59] Morrison J. 'Left behind'North of the border? Economic disadvantage and intersectional inequalities in post-pandemic Scotland. Scottish Affairs. Scotland. 2022;**31**(4):393-418

[60] Kuramochi I, Iwayama T, Brandt C, Yoshimasu H, Bien CG, Hagemann A. Assessment of self-stigma in epilepsy: Validation of the German version epilepsy self-stigma scale (ESSS-G). Epilepsia Open. 2023;**8**(2):946-958

[61] Makhado L, Maphula A, Makhado TG, Musekwa OP. Perspective chapter: Practical approaches to enhance successful lives among people living with epilepsy. Health and Educational Success-Recent Perspectives. 2022. DOI: 10.5772/intechopen.106649

[62] Makhado TG, Lebese RT, Maputle MS. Development and validation of epilepsy life skills guidelines for primary school learners and teachers in Limpopo and Mpumalanga provinces. Children. 2023;**10**(7):1194

[63] Fisher K, Desroches ML, Marsden D, Rees S, Northway R, Horan P, et al. International nursing actions to reduce health inequities faced by people with intellectual and developmental disability. Online Journal of Issues in Nursing. 2022;**27**(3). DOI: 10.3912/OJIN.Vol27No03Man07

[64] Alabi OT, Musbau LA, Wojujutari AK, Abiola SS, Chioma OC. Relationship between psychological distress and perceived stigma on mental well-being in people with epilepsy: Self-compassion as a moderator. Arab Journal of Psychiatry. 2023;**34**(1):56-63

[65] Coleman H, Peterson CL, Walker C. Understanding the experiences of stigma in relation to social support among an Australian community cohort of people living with epilepsy. Australian Journal of Social Issues. 2022;**57**(4):920-937

[66] Evett D, Hutchinson K, Bierbaum M, Perikic N, Proctor C, Rapport F, et al. Peer support and social network groups among people living with epilepsy: A scoping review. Epilepsy & Behavior. 2021;**124**:108381

[67] Shawahna R. Agreement of Palestinian nursing students with recommendations to eliminate epilepsy stigma and change perception of the general public about epilepsy: A cross-sectional study. Epilepsy & Behavior. 2020;**109**:107126

[68] Giuliano L, Cicero CE, Padilla S, Camargo M, Sofia V, Zappia M, et al. Knowledge and attitudes towards epilepsy among nonmedical health workers in rural Bolivia: Results after a long-term activity in the Chaco region. Epilepsy & Behavior. 2018;**85**:58-63

[69] Mariga L, McConkey R. Inclusive Education in Low-Income Countries: A Resource Book for Teacher Educators, Parent Trainers and Community Development. African Books Collective; 2014

[70] Kirsh B, Krupa T, Luong D. How do supervisors perceive and manage employee mental health issues in their workplaces? Work. 2018;**59**(4):547-555

[71] Heijnders M, Van Der Meij S. The fight against stigma: An overview of stigma-reduction strategies and

interventions. Psychology, Health & Medicine. 2006;**11**(3):353-363

[72] Lorenzo T, van Pletzen E, Booyens M. Determining the competences of community based workers for disability-inclusive development in rural areas of South Africa, Botswana and Malawi. Rural and Remote Health. 2015;**15**(2):62-75

[73] World Health Organization. CureAll Framework: WHO Global Initiative for Childhood Cancer: Increasing Access, Advancing Quality, Saving Lives. World Health Organization. 2021. Licence: CC BY-NC-SA 3.0 IGO. Available from: https://creativecommons.org/licenses/by-nc-sa/3.0/igo/

[74] Mpofu J, Sefotho MM, Maree JG. Psychological well-being of adolescents with physical disabilities in Zimbabwean inclusive community settings: An exploratory study. African Journal of Disability. 2017;**6**:1-7

Chapter 8

Perspective Chapter: Determinants of Health-Care Seeking Behaviors and Quality of Life in Children with Epilepsy in Nigeria

Sylvia Tochukwu Echendu, Ngozi N. Joe-Ikechebelu, Amalachukwu O. Odita, Esther N. Umeadi, Njideka C. Uchefuna, Wilson C. Igwe, Izunna S. Okwelogu and Chinonye V. Iloanya

Abstract

Epilepsy is the commonest neurological condition affecting every sphere of a child's life ranging from physical and cognitive performances, and mixed feelings for the affected family. These feelings are worsened by the cultural beliefs, myths, and stigmatization that surround epilepsy with a consequent reduction in the healthcare-seeking behaviors and quality of life of these children. The goal of management is to control seizures with minimal use of antiepileptic medications and to improve the child's quality of life. This work is aimed to understand the health-seeking behavior of families and children diagnosed with epilepsy in Nigeria, the factors that influence their decisions, and the need to plan a "need-based" comprehensive healthcare program for all stakeholders, particularly the disprivileged groups. Despite some improvement in access to healthcare in Nigeria, there are existing inequalities relative to culture, socioeconomic class, accessibility to universal health insurance, and gender. Knowledge of barriers to optimal healthcare-seeking behavior could help reduce the impact of epilepsy on children's development and consequently improved quality of life. Efforts should be made to educate children with epilepsy, their caregivers, and other affected stakeholders and periodic trainings organized for the health workers. Subsidizing the cost of care by support groups and government is vital.

Keywords: epilepsy, pediatrics, determinants, health-seeking, quality

1. Introduction

Epilepsy is a chronic non-communicable disorder of the brain characterized by recurrent unprovoked seizures with neurological, cognitive, psychological, and social consequences [1]. The International League against epilepsy requires at least two unprovoked seizures occurring greater than 24 hours apart or one unprovoked seizure and the probability of further seizures occurring over the next 10 years, or the presence of an epilepsy syndrome to make a definitive diagnosis of epilepsy [2]. It is the most common neurological disorder in children and sometimes has a negative impact on the quality of life of affected children [3, 4]. The mortality rate in people affected by epilepsy is 2–4 times higher than the rest of the population and 5–10 times higher in children [5]. Therefore, epilepsy affects the quality of life significantly because of its chronicity, frequent seizures, needs for regular medications, side effects of the medications, epilepsy-related injuries, and stigmatization surrounding it. The traditional medical goal in the management of epilepsy is aimed to control the seizure. However, current practices have moved further into improving the quality of life of these patients.

Appropriate healthcare-seeking behavior toward epilepsy can reduce its morbidity and mortality rate and ultimately improve the quality of life of those affected [6]. On the other hand, poor health-seeking behavior is a major bane in the outcome of seizure management and eventually the effect of seizures on the quality of life of children with epilepsy (CWE) in Nigeria and many low- and medium-income countries (LMIC).

2. Determinants of healthcare-seeking behavior

2.1 Caregiver perception

Children with epilepsy (CWE) just like other children are dependent on their caregivers and so the caregiver's perception and belief systems with regards to seizure etiology (hereditary, influence of spirits and witchcraft, excessive intake of palm oil) and their cultural background influence decisions regarding the choice of care for them [7–11]. In many parts of Nigeria, epilepsy is considered a spiritual disease and not amenable to medical treatment, consequently, treatment choices are often unorthodox involving consultation with traditional and spiritual healers [7, 11–13]. Sometimes herbal therapies are readily available at home and serve as the first treatment option before presentation to other facilities [7].

2.2 Myths and misconceptions about epilepsy

Misconceptions about the cause of epilepsy, mode of spread, and preferred mode of treatment play a significant role in the management of children with epilepsy in Nigeria [14]. In some parts of Nigeria particularly in rural settings, people perceive that epilepsy is a curse by the gods, a sign of witchcraft activity, or demon possession. In such communities, epilepsy is regarded as a spiritual problem that is not amenable to medical treatment, so a traditional or spiritual approach to treatment is often the first or preferred option [8, 12, 15]. These include scarifications, herbal preparations, spiritual exorcism, charms, fire/smoke therapy, and sometimes sacrificial offerings. Igwe et al. in South East Nigeria reported that the major reason for patronizing unorthodox medical practitioners was a belief in the care, its affordability, and perception of the cause of the disease [7]. Sometimes, the patients eventually present to the hospital when the seizures persist/worsen or when they develop complications.

2.3 Finances: Cost of care

The availability and affordability of medical care cost influence the health-seeking behaviors of caregivers of children with epilepsy (CWE) [7]. A recent survey reveals that about 97% of the Nigerian population does not have any form of health insurance, inevitably, the additional financial burden of epilepsy care is usually borne by the caregiver [16]. Furthermore, an estimated population of 88.4 million people in Nigeria reportedly live in extreme poverty (on less than 1.90 US dollars a day) and accounted for 12.9% of extremely poor people globally in 2022 [17]. Consequently, cost of care and proximity to care are important factors that influence healthcare-seeking behaviors in Nigeria. These out-of-pocket costs and productivity losses can create substantial burdens on households. The consequence is a decline in the demand for healthcare services, poor compliance with therapy, seizure recurrence, and the increased patronage of quacks or outright abandonment of the children to a profoundly diminished quality of life. In addition, there can be deprivation of socioeconomic materiality and resources to other family members, deepening the family's financial crises.

2.4 Parental level of education

Parental level of education and in particular, the maternal level of education is a major determinant of health-seeking behavior. In Ibadan, Lagunju et al. reported a statistically significant association between maternal educational level, economic agency, and the health-related quality of life (HRQOL), with children of mothers with less than 10 years of formal education having a poorer HRQOL [18]. With the higher educational level of parents, the potential for the affected child's parents to seek appropriate care early has been linked to high prognostic factors. Whereas less educated parents may not have a robust understanding of the chronic nature of the illness or the need to adhere to therapy and follow-up assessment throughout the course of treatment. Children from less educated backgrounds have a greater risk of lower drug compliance, relapses, refractory seizures, and drop-out of therapy. This is because as minors, they depend on their caregiver's perception and cooperation for decisions that affect them including medical treatment. Besides, educated caregivers are more likely to seek care early and from orthodox practitioners than uneducated caregivers who are less compliant with medications and counseling. The work done by Igwe et al. [7] also confirmed these findings.

2.5 Role of teachers

For children that attend school, there is the risk of having seizures in school and at such times, the knowledge and attitudes of their teachers come to play in determining the kind of care the CWE get before their parents are reached. In addition, in rural settings, some parents consider teachers quite knowledgeable and can easily be influenced by their suggestions [15]. In some surveys in different sub-regions in Nigeria, the knowledge of teachers was surprisingly low and many opted for alternative medicine as the preferred mode of care of epilepsy [11, 13, 19, 20].

2.6 Stigmatization

The stigmatization associated with epilepsy in many parts of Nigeria also affects healthcare-seeking behaviors as some parents, especially in pastoral settings are reticent to seek treatment for seizures in hospitals for fear of getting the "epilepsy" label which impacts negatively the family name and may be an obstacle for marriage of ladies in their families. They choose rather to seek help with alternative healthcare personnel where other factors such as "spiritual attack" are attributed to the cause of the illness [6, 7]. This is further accentuated by efforts of family members in certain Nigerian cultural groups (like the Igbos in the South-east) to maintain the "chastity" of their family lines and avoid impurity with dreaded diseases like epilepsy [15]. For this reason, there is often resistance to marriage to any relation to a known person living with epilepsy which results in secretiveness and shrouding of disease notification.

2.7 Health workers' knowledge and approach

Healthcare professionals are motivators of health and healthcare-seeking behaviors of patients. Often, patients relinquish the choice of care concerning their health to the doctors and other healthcare professionals believing that they are knowledgeable. However, concerning epilepsy and the myths and prejudices girding it, a study done in South East, Nigeria among healthcare professionals (doctors from different specialties and nurses) reported poor knowledge of epilepsy among health workers. In the study, only about 50% of doctors <10 yrs and 51.2% >10 yrs. had training in pediatric epilepsy [21]. Further, the study also showed their reluctance to undergo the training [21]. Physicians with poor knowledge of the pediatric epilepsy have little or nothing to step down to the public and accordingly, the patients and their caregiver gets little or no information concerning epilepsy from their physicians.

- All these factors determine not only the health-seeking behavior of parents of children with epilepsy but also affect the timing between the onset of seizures to the time of presentation to specialist care. Igwe et al. reported that only about 45% presented within 6 months while about 26% presented within 2 years [7]. Within the period when they have not presented to the specialists, several unorthodox practices are employed at home and other traditional facilities based on the religious and cultural beliefs and perceptions of the disease. Late presentation increases morbidity, decreases the quality of life, and consequently, the mortality rate in these children with epilepsy is increased.

3. Quality of life (QOL) of children with epilepsy in Nigeria

The World Health Organization (WHO) defines Quality of life (QOL) as "an individual's perception of their position in life in the context of the culture and value systems in which they live and in relation to their pretensions, prospects, norms, and concerns" [22]. Many chronic disorders such as epilepsy, cerebral palsy, or sickle cell anemia are known to have profound negative effects on the quality of life of the patients and their families. They may cause several changes in almost all spheres of the child's life, from self-care, self-image, and daily duties to emotional and cognitive performance and relationships with their peers. The new trend in the management of most chronic conditions is not only to control the disease but to improve the quality of life of the patients and to ensure that patients live optimally to their satisfaction as this will help improve compliance with medications and follow-up. In Nigeria, in particular, studies across different geopolitical regions have shown that epilepsy reduces the quality of life of affected individuals significantly [18, 23–25]. The same applies in some other low- and middle-income countries [26–28]. Conversely, Aldenkamp in a study in the Netherlands reported a high quality of life (QOL) for a majority of the patients studied. Nevertheless, those patients had uncomplicated well-controlled epilepsy [29]. This underscores the importance of bridging the treatment gap and optimizing seizure control among children living with epilepsy as this will markedly improve their health-related quality of life.

Factors that contribute to the low quality of life in children with epilepsy in Nigeria include poor health-seeking behaviors, seizure frequency, stigma, availability and accessibility to health facilities, availability of drugs, adverse drug reactions, quality of medical care, parental level of education, rural residence, the attitude of health workers, affordability of medical care cost, seizure frequency, polytherapy, adverse drug reactions (ADRs) to antiepileptic medications (AEDs), and duration of epilepsy [23, 30].

Many children living with epilepsy face the scourge of stigmatization regularly particularly female children due to the erroneous belief that epilepsy is contagious and can be transmitted through contact with affected individuals or their body products such as saliva, urine, and feces of the affected individuals [8, 11]. They are sometimes restrained from interacting with others and those with refractory seizures are sometimes withdrawn from school. Unfortunately, in certain situations, they are outrightly rejected by the school authorities. For example, Nuhu et al. reported an 18% school rejection rate among a group of adolescents with epilepsy in Kaduna, a megacity in North Central Nigeria [25]. This is mostly due to the perceived or even experienced stigma associated with circumstances of seizures in public places and the risk of physical injuries as well as the attitude of teachers to them [15].

The Nigerian child has a right to education as enshrined in Chapter 2 of the 1999 Constitution of the Federal Republic of Nigeria and the Child's Rights Act of 2003 [31]. This is important because quality education can impact appreciatively on the quality of life of a child with short- and long-term benefits. In Ibadan, Lagunju [18] reported a statistically significant association between maternal level of education and impaired health-related quality of life (HRQOL) such that children of mothers with lower than secondary education have a poorer HRQOL. But uncontrolled epilepsy robs a child of their fundamental right to education and this can be attributed to several factors such as uncontrolled seizures resulting in absenteeism, stigmatization in school, and the adverse effects of some anti-seizure medications on cognition [25, 32]. In a 5-year study in the University teaching hospital, Ibadan, Lagunju et al. reported that 10.6% had severe to profound limitations in school work, 6.1% dropped out of school on account of severe epilepsy, 36.4% missed school occasionally as a result of seizures, 18.3% had deterioration in academic performance while 53.0% of the children did not experience any form of limitation in school work [18].

The impact of epilepsy extends beyond those affected by seizures to other members of the family particularly parents who are likely to witness anxiety, passions of helplessness, or guilt in response to the child's seizures and seizure-threat. Sometimes, these factors can lead to a shattered cohesion in the family union and eventually a divorce. In view of this, parental emotional stability has been found a major predictor of the quality of life in children with epilepsy, and psychopathology in parents is significantly associated with poorer quality of life of these adolescents [33].

Epilepsy is an illness that has a major impact on the HRQOL of Nigerian children, with significant impairments in at least one-quarter of the cases in all the disciplines tested among patients presenting in a tertiary health institution in South West

Nigeria [18]. The duration of epilepsy, seizure frequency, and severity, number of antiepileptic drugs (polytherapy), and adverse drug reactions (ADRs) to antiepileptic drugs (AED) are significantly associated with poor QOL in adolescents with epilepsy [33]. On the other hand, epilepsy can be controlled in a large number of cases so it is advocated that children with epilepsy get the right treatment early. Usually, the goal of treatment is to achieve complete resolution of seizure or a significant reduction in seizure frequency with a minimal number of drugs as well as to ensure the best quality of life for the child [18]. Therefore appropriate treatment should be instituted early and heavy polytherapy as well as specific medications with severe cognitive adverse effects should be avoided.

Seizures are often associated with comorbidities that affect the quality of life of sufferers, particularly for patients with early-onset seizures, status seizures, and long stays before presentation in the hospital for care. These include cerebral palsy, visual impairment, hemiplegia, attention deficit hyperactivity disorder, irrational behavior, auditory disability, visual disability, expressive aphasia, intellectual disability (mental retardation), deafness, etc. [34–36]. Akinsulore et al. also reported psychiatric comorbidities such as depressive disorders, anxiety disorders, disruptive behaviors, and personality disorders in adolescents with epilepsy [33].

Due to the myriads of health and social problems that children with epilepsy present with, a multi-disciplinary management approach involving pediatric neurologists, ophthalmologists, ear, nose, and throat surgeons, speech therapists, psychologists, physiotherapists, and social workers, becomes imperative and pivotal. They are often depressed and unhappy with their lives being dependent on drugs and frequent hospital visitations and also not being free to mingle with other children. Efforts should be geared toward reducing the number of anti-epileptic medications as poly-pharmacy significantly reduces compliance and consequently contributes to poor quality of life seen in children with epilepsy.

Education plays a key role in the management of children with epilepsy and should involve the child, the parents, and society at large. Accurate information should be given concerning the cause, consequences, self management, epilepsy's risks including injuries, other morbidities and mortalities, skill development, and available support groups and resources within and around their environ. They should also be supported to go to school because education improves compliance with medications and quality of care. Enlightenment campaigns against the myth surrounding epilepsy and societal stigma should be paramount.

4. Conclusion

Epilepsy is a neurologic condition surrounded by myths and consequently, stigmatization. It present not only with seizures but also with other comorbidities with a resultant reduction in the quality of life of these patients. Efforts should be made to educate the general public including personnel on the cause and management of children with epilepsy.

Acknowledgements

Great thanks to all that in one way or the other contributed to the success of this work from conception to its final form.

Funding

There was no direct nor indirect funding, received for this work.

Authors' contribution

All authors were involved in the conception, writing, and revision of the manuscript. All authors read and approved the final manuscript.

Competing interests

The authors declare no competing interests.

Author details

Sylvia Tochukwu Echendu[1,4*], Ngozi N. Joe-Ikechebelu[2,4], Amalachukwu O. Odita[1,3], Esther N. Umeadi[1,3], Njideka C. Uchefuna[1], Wilson C. Igwe[1,3], Izunna S. Okwelogu[4,5] and Chinonye V. Iloanya[4]

1 Department of Paediatrics, Nnamdi Azikiwe University Teaching Hospital, Nigeria

2 Chukwuemeka Odumegwu Ojukwu University Teaching Hospital, Awka, Nigeria

3 Department of paediatric Nnamdi Azikiwe University, Awka, Nigeria

4 Life International Hospital, Awka, Nigeria

5 Department of Parasitology And Entomology Nnamdi Azikiwe University, Awka, Nigeria

*Address all correspondence to: sylvianpc2015@gmail.com

References

[1] Sarmast ST, Abdullahi AM, Jahan N. Current Classification of Seizures and Epilepsies: Scope, Limitations and Recommendations for Future Action. Cureus; 2020;**12**(9):1-17. DOI: 10.7759/cureus.10549

[2] Fisher RS, Acevedo C, Arzimanoglou A, Bogacz A, Cross JH, Elger CE, et al. ILAE official report: A practical clinical definition of epilepsy. Epilepsia. 2014;**55**(4):475-482

[3] Aronu A, Uwaezuoke N, Chinawa J, Bisi-Onyemaechi A, Ojinnaka N. Health-related quality of life in children and adolescents with epilepsy in Enugu: Need for targeted intervention. Nigerian Journal of Clinical Practice. 2021;**24**(4):517-524

[4] Fine A, Wirrell EC. Seizures in children. Pediatrics in Review. 2020;**41**(7):321-347

[5] Minardi C, Minacapelli R, Valastro P, Vasile F, Pitino S, Pavone P, et al. Epilepsy in children: From diagnosis to treatment with focus on emergency. Journal of Clinical Medicine. 2019;**8**(1):39. DOI: 103390/jcm8010039

[6] Ojinnaka N, C, Aronu AE, Ojinnaka GC, Uwaezuoke NA, Bisi-Onyemaechi AI. Health-seeking behavior of care-givers of children with epilepsy in a resource-poor country. Acta Scientific Neurology. 2019;**2**(2):1-5

[7] Igwe WC, Umeadi EN, Echendu ST, Odita AO. Sociodemographic factors influencing health care–seeking behavior for pediatric epilepsy in Southeast Nigeria. Journal of Neurosciences in Rural Practice. 2022;**13**:448-452

[8] Ekeh BC, Ekrikpo UE. The knowledge, attitude, and perception towards epilepsy amongst medical students in Uyo, Southern Nigeria. Advances in Medicine. 2015;**2015**:1-6

[9] Ademilokun TF, Agunbiade OM. Aetiological explanations of epilepsy and implications on treatments options among Yoruba traditional healers in Southwest Nigeria. African Sociological Review. 2021;**25**(1):86-111

[10] Osungbade KO, Siyanbade SL. Myths, misconceptions, and misunderstandings about epilepsy in a Nigerian rural community: Implications for community health interventions. Epilepsy & Behavior. 2011;**21**(4):425-429

[11] Sanya EO, Salami TAT, Goodman OO, Buhari OIN, Araoye MO. Perception and attitude to epilepsy among teachers in primary, secondary and tertiary educational institutions in middle belt Nigeria. Tropical Doctor. 2005;**35**(3):153-156

[12] Okunola P, Nwaneri D. A study on childhood epilepsy among traders in Benin City Nigeria. Nigerian Medical Journal. 2019;**60**(4):175-180

[13] Owolabi LF, Shehu NM, Owolabi SD. Epilepsy and Education in developing countries: a survey of school teachers' knowledge about epilepsy and their attitude towards students with epilepsy in Northwestern Nigeria. Pan African Medical Journal. 2014;**18**:255. DOI: 10.11604/pamj.2014.18.255.3607

[14] Flying Doctors Nigeria. Is epilepsy a spiritual problem? Available from: https://www.flyingdoctorsnigeria.com/2018/05/08/is-epilepsy-a-spiritual-problem/. 2018

[15] Ezeala-Adikaibe BA, Achor JU, Aneke E, Ijoma U, Onodugo OD, Orjioke C, et al. Pattern and determinants of self-reported enacted stigma among rural dwellers living with epilepsy attending a tertiary health facility in Enugu State Nigeria. Seizure. 2018;**56**:60-66

[16] Akokuwebe ME, Idemudia ES. A comparative cross-sectional study of the prevalence and determinants of health insurance coverage in Nigeria and South Africa: A multi-country analysis of demographic health surveys. International Journal of Environmental Research and Public Health. 2022;**19**(3):1766. DOI: 10.3390/ijerph19031766

[17] Sasu D, D. People living in extreme poverty in Nigeria 2016-2022, by gender. Statista. 2003. Available from: http://www.statista.Com. Accessed june 10, 2023

[18] Lagunju I, Akinyinka OO, Adebola EO, Akinbami FO, Brown BJ, Olorundare E, et al. Health-related quality of life of Nigerian children with epilepsy. African Journal of Neurological Sciences. 2009;**28**(1):23-36

[19] Mustapha A, Odu O, Akande O. Knowledge, attitudes and perceptions of epilepsy among secondary school teachers in Osogbo South-West Nigeria: A community based study. Nigerian Journal of Clinical Practice. 2013;**16**(1):12

[20] Ojinnaka NC. Teachers' perception of epilepsy in Nigeria: A community-based study. Seizure. 2002;**11**(6):386-391

[21] Igwe WC, Umeadi EN, Echendu ST, Odita AO, Anyabolu EN. Primary care physicians knowledge and approach to paediatric epilepsy care in Nnamdi Azikiwe University Teaching Hospital, Nnewi. International Journal of Biomedical Research. 2021;**12**:e5674. DOI: 10.7439/ijbr.v12i10.5674

[22] WHOQOL. User manual Programme on mental health division of mental health and prevention of substance abuse World Health Organization [Internet]. [cited 2023 May 5]. Available from: https://www.who.int/toolkits/whoqol

[23] Gbiri CA, Akingbohungbe AD. Determinants of quality of life in Nigerian children and adolescents with epilepsy: A hospital-based study. Disability, CBR & Inclusive Development. 2012;**22**(3):89-93

[24] Onwuekwe IO, Onodugo OD, Ezeala-Adikaibe B, Aguwa EN, Ejim EC, Ndukuba K, et al. Pattern and presentation of epilepsy in Nigerian Africans: A study of trends in the Southeast. Transactions of the Royal Society of Tropical Medicine and Hygiene. 2009;**103**(8):785-789

[25] Nuhu FT, Yusuf AJ, Sheikh TL, Eseigbe EE. Poor academic performance among adolescents with epilepsy in Kaduna, Northern Nigeria: A case-control study. South African Journal of Child Health. 2012;**6**(4):132-134

[26] Minwuyelet F, Mulugeta H, Tsegaye D, Lake B, Getie A, Tsegaye B, et al. Quality of life and associated factors among patients with epilepsy at specialized hospitals, Northwest Ethiopia; 2019. PLoS One. 2022;**17**(1):e0262814

[27] Gholami A, Salarilak S, Lotfabadi P, Kiani F, Rajabi A, Mansori K, et al. Quality of life in epileptic patients compared with healthy people. Medical Journal of the Islamic Republic of Iran. 2016;**30**:388. Available from: https://mjiri.iums.ac.ir

[28] Kinyanjui DW, Kathuku DM, Mburu JM. Quality of life among

patients living with epilepsy attending the neurology clinic at Kenyatta national hospital, Nairobi, Kenya: A comparative study. Health and Quality of Life Outcomes. 2013;**11**(1):98. DOI: 10.1186/1477-7523-11-98

[29] Aldenkamp AP, Van Donselaar CA, Flamman H, Lafarre DLW. Psychosocial reactions to the epilepsy in an unselected group of patients with epilepsy under treatment in general hospitals. Seizure. 2003;**12**(2):101-106

[30] Igwe W. Challenges in the management of pediatric epilepsy in Nigeria. Tropical Journal of Medical Research. 2016;**19**(1):1. DOI. 10.4103/1119-0388.172063

[31] Magbadelo JO. Children's rights to education and wellbeing in Nigeria. World Affairs: The Journal of International Issues. 2023;**23**(1):112-127

[32] Ijff DM, Aldenkamp AP. Cognitive side-effects of antiepileptic drugs in children. In: Handbook of Clinical Neurology, Elsevier, Netherlands. 2013;**111**(73):707-718

[33] Akinsulore A, Adewuya A. Psychosocial aspects of epilepsy in Nigeria: A review. African Journal of Psychiatry (Johannesbg). 2010;**13**:351-356

[34] Eyong KI, Ekanem EE, Asindi AA, Chimaeze T. Clinical profile of childhood epilepsy in Nigerian children seen in a tertiary hospital. International Journal of Contemporary Pediatrics. 2017;**4**(4):1138-1141

[35] Iloeje SO. The pattern of childhood epilepsy with mental retardation in Nigeria. Journal of Tropical Pediatrics. 1989;**35**(4):163-168

[36] Ojuawo A, Joiner KT. Childhood epilepsy in Ilorin, Nigeria. East African Medical Journal. 1997;**74**(2):72-75

Chapter 9

Perspective Chapter: How Can We Provide Lifelong Support for People with Epilepsy to Reduce Their Self-Stigma?

Izumi Kuramochi, Takayuki Iwayama and Sakie Shimotsu

Abstract

Self-stigma denotes the internalization of negative societal attitudes, and it is commonly referred in patients with epilepsy (PWE). Higher levels of self-stigma have been linked to lower self-esteem. According to the author's research, there is no significant correlation between knowledge level and self-stigma among PWE, and short-term treatment to control seizures alone proves inadequate for reducing self-stigma. These findings provide insights into the enduring nature of self-stigmatization, which appears to be influenced by cultural background, environmental factors, and personal experiences. Firstly, rectifying misinformation is crucial, as it promotes critical thinking and challenges cultural shame rather than accepting it. Secondly, cognitive approaches can be beneficial in helping individuals identify and overcome self-stigmatizing attitudes and beliefs. Recognizing the presence of social stigma and self-stigma are instrumental in reducing self-stigma. Lastly, facilitating individuals fostering a sense of agency in their lives can be accomplished through decision-making and empowerment strategies. Assisting clients in identifying their strengths and enabling them to make autonomous life choices can foster improved self-esteem and decrease self-stigma. While the primary goal of epilepsy treatment is the reduction of seizures, it is crucial for all stakeholders to acknowledge the persistent nature of self-stigma throughout the lifelong treatment trajectory of PWE.

Keywords: epilepsy, prejudice, self-stigma, quality of life, epilepsy self-stigma scale

1. Introduction

When considering "epilepsy," individuals often form mental associations or stereotypes about this medical condition. Stereotypes are constructed and established based on the prevailing social characteristics of the majority within a specific society, generally accepted as factual by most individuals in that society [1]. When individuals endorse negative stereotypes, it develops negative emotions and emotional responses, commonly known as "prejudice." For instance, someone who believes that people with epilepsy (PWE) pose a danger may experience fear toward individuals with this condition. The issue received significant attention in Japan following the media's extensive coverage of traffic accidents involving individuals with epilepsy in 2011. As a result, the association between the public image of epilepsy and the concept of danger became more pronounced in 2013 [2].

These emotional reactions can manifest as discrimination, the behavioral response of harboring negative thoughts and feelings toward stigmatized groups. Due to fear (prejudice) and the acceptance of the associated stereotype, the general public may opt to maintain a physical and emotional distance from individuals with epilepsy. Epilepsy-related stigma is prevalent in numerous cultures [3, 4] and is widely recognized as one of the most significant factors negatively impacting the lives of PWE and their families [5–8].

Among those who feel "stigmatized" by society and live within that society are PWE themselves. Some PWE has stereotypes and self-stigmas about themselves. These include acceptance of self-stereotypes (e.g., "I am a danger to myself with epileptic seizures."), prejudice (e.g., "I am afraid of myself"), and the accompanying self-discrimination (e.g., social isolation due to self-blame). Internalizing negative stereotypes can trigger adverse emotional reactions, such as low self-esteem and diminished self-efficacy. Self-discrimination, particularly self-isolation, has detrimental effects, including reduced healthcare utilization, poorer health outcomes, and decreased quality of life [9]. Low self-efficacy and self-esteem have also been associated with missed opportunities for employment and independent living [10, 11]. Link et al. referred to this as the modified labeling theory, highlighting that individuals who internalize the stigma of mental illness worsen their condition due to the harm caused by internalized experiences [12, 13]. Self-stigmatization entails a reduction in self-worth and a detrimental impact on one's aspirations toward personal goals. Consequently, self-stigma emerges as an intrapersonal phenomenon that leads to adverse health outcomes and diminishes the quality of life experienced by individuals diagnosed with epilepsy (PWE) [9, 14].

2. Efforts to reduce the stigma of epilepsy

Epilepsy has been documented as far back as 4000 B.C. and has had severe physical, mental, and social effects on patients for centuries, with no difference in age, race, country, or geographical location [15]. In response to the history of prejudice due to lack of knowledge, preconceptions, and discrimination against epilepsy, in 1997, the International Epilepsy Congress and the WHO, in collaboration with the International League Against Epilepsy (ILAE) and the International Bureau of Epilepsy (IBE), launched an international campaign called "Out of the (Shadows [16]).

The Intersectoral Global Action Plan (IGAP) on epilepsy and other neurological disorders aims to enhance accessibility to care and treatment for people with neurological disorders while concurrently preventing new cases and advocating brain health and development throughout the lifespan [17]. This comprehensive initiative spans 10 years, from 2022 to 2031. Its approval by 193 states on 27 May during the 75th World Health Assembly [17] signifies a decade-long commitment to prioritizing brain health by bolstering policy focus and governance; facilitating effective and timely diagnosis, treatment, and care; implementing strategies for promotion and prevention; fostering research and innovation; and fortifying information systems, as well as enhancing the public health approach to epilepsy [18]. However, to mitigate the societal stigma associated with epilepsy, continued efforts will be necessary to sustain the campaign's impact.

3. Lifelong support for epilepsy patients to reduce self-stigma

What approaches help reduce self-stigma among people with epilepsy?

To adequately facilitate the reduction of self-stigma, it is imperative to comprehend the intricacies involved in the formation of self-stigma within distinct cultural contexts. The authors have investigated the actual status of self-stigma in epilepsy patients in Japan, developed a measurement scale, and conducted group psychoeducation programs [19–21]. This paper therefore introduces the studies conducted by the authors and discusses the direction of clinical practice and future research aimed at reducing self-stigma in Japan.

3.1 Self-stigma among epilepsy patients (results of qualitative analysis study)

The authors used semi-structured interviews and their qualitative analysis to analyze elements of self-stigma among Japanese PWE [19]. For historical reasons, epilepsy in Japan is treated by neurology, neurosurgery, and neuropsychiatry. In Japan's administrative classification, epilepsy is classified as a psychiatric disorder, necessitating the involvement of psychiatrists due to its distinctive features. Analysis of 206 verbatim data obtained from epilepsy patients attending outpatient clinics in Japan resulted in the extraction of 74 codes. Qualitative analysis of these codes identified 22 subcategories of epilepsy-related self-stigma and three major categories: self-stigma, perceived social stigma, and actual distress/troubles. The subsequent paragraphs provide a detailed description of the self-stigma categories derived from the qualitative analysis.

Concerning self-stigma among PWE, negative beliefs are not only negative cognitions about the disease and diagnosis of epilepsy, such as "I am not capable" and "I am a weak person," but also "I have an image that epileptic seizures are something that makes me foam and fall" and "I will be a burden to others if I have an epileptic seizure." It was found that these included negative perceptions about epileptic seizures, such as "I will be a burden to others" and "People will feel uncomfortable if they figure out I have epileptic seizures."

The findings additionally revealed the presence of "negative feelings about epileptic seizures," exemplified by expressions such as "I do not want to have an epileptic seizure because I will burst into a bubble and collapse" and "It is painful to be seen having an epileptic seizure." Furthermore, sentiments such as "It is embarrassing to be seen having an epileptic seizure," "I hate going to a psychiatrist," and "I have an aversion to seeing a psychiatrist" were also expressed within the dataset. Influenced by these adverse emotional experiences, the patients conveyed challenges encompassing various aspects of the disclosure, including "difficulties in revealing my epilepsy diagnosis to others," "challenges in disclosing my condition to my family," "obstacles in informing my teachers about my epilepsy," "struggles in divulging my epilepsy diagnosis to my workplace," and "difficulties in communicating my condition to doctors from other medical departments," among others. The respondents admitted to behavioral changes such as "difficulty in telling my family that I have epilepsy," "wanting to hide the fact that I have epilepsy," "not wanting to take my medication in public," and "wanting to hide the fact that I have epilepsy and have to go to the hospital for treatment."

The behavioral manifestations of these negative changes were identified to be more prominently evident within the cognitive component, characterized by a "negative evaluation of my life so far," as opposed to the emotional component, which featured a "decreased general self-confidence." Additionally, the negative behavioral changes, precisely the "abandonment of various activities due to the presence of epilepsy," exhibited a lesser degree of recognition compared to the cognitive component.

These findings specifically examine the stigma of epilepsy in Japan, and it is crucial to note that not all of the identified factors may be applicable to other countries or cultures. In particular, the pronounced association with psychiatry may be influenced by the distinctive medical context of Japan. However, those individuals involved in epilepsy care need to acknowledge that patients with epilepsy may experience and endure these self-stigmas associated with the condition.

3.2 Creation of the epilepsy self-stigma scale

The Epilepsy Self-Stigma Scale (ESSS) [21] (**Table 1**) was developed to measure self-stigma explicitly pertaining to "epilepsy" and to provide a convenient assessment scale suitable for use in a short consultation time. The development of the ESSS involved the utilization of results from qualitative analysis in Japan. Subsequently, the questionnaire was formulated based on the results of a qualitative analysis, and an exploratory factor analysis was conducted based on data obtained from 100 epilepsy patients attending outpatient clinics at multiple medical institutions. As a result, a final questionnaire comprising three factors (Internalization of stigma, Societal incomprehension, and Confidentiality) and eight items was derived. The ESSS items are rated on a four-point Likert-type scale: 1: Strongly Disagree, 2: Slightly agree, 3: Agree, 4: Strongly Agree. Total scores range from 8 to 32. The higher the total score, the greater is the extent of the self-stigma toward epilepsy. The calculation of scores for each factor enables a comprehensive assessment of the relative significance of different dimensions of self-stigma. In addition, high internal consistency has been obtained across the entire scale and all subscales, and high retest reliability and adequate construct validity concerning depressive symptoms

	Disagree	Weakly Agree	Agree	Strongly Agree
1. When I hear news about traffic accidents related to epileptic seizures, I feel like I am being told about myself.	1	2	3	4
2. I feel discriminated against by others because of epilepsy.	1	2	3	4
3. I sometimes feel embarrassed about epilepsy.	1	2	3	4
4. I feel different from others because I have epilepsy.	1	2	3	4
5. Ordinary people do not understand my suffering from epilepsy and the worry of seizures.	1	2	3	4
6. Few people have the correct information about the disease of epilepsy.	1	2	3	4
7. It is hard to tell others that I have epilepsy.	1	2	3	4
8. I want to hide the fact that I go to the hospital to receive therapy for epilepsy.	1	2	3	4

This questionnaire will ask you about what you think about having epilepsy.
For each question, please choose the most appropriate number from the scale to the right of each sentence.

Table 1.
Epilepsy self-stigma scale (eight items) [21].

and self-esteem. Cronbach's α for the total scale and each factor demonstrated good internal consistency (α = 0.76–0.87). The ESSS has undergone a prolonged development process, and its utilization in various studies has been relatively limited, resulting in a scarcity of comprehensive information. However, it is noteworthy that no significant correlation was observed between external criteria, such as an objective assessment of self-stigma conducted by the subject's physician, and the total score on the ESSS, which contrasts with findings from comparable scales. This finding aligns with the conceptualization of self-stigma as internalized stigma and highlights the challenge of accurately assessing a patient's self-stigma solely within the consultation setting.

3.3 Efforts to reduce self-stigma in people with epilepsy

3.3.1 Educational needs, psychosocial education programs

The first step in reducing self-stigma is to provide accurate information about PWE and its supporters. Education and awareness can reduce misconceptions and prejudices about epilepsy and promote public understanding and empathy. Education should be targeted not only to PWE and others affected by the disease but also to the general public, teachers, and healthcare professionals. People with epilepsy must understand their condition and learn about appropriate treatment and daily living precautions.

Psychosocial education programs on epilepsy have been conducted in various countries, and their usefulness has been reported [22]. Although psychosocial and educational programs took many forms depending on the country and context in which they were implemented, most interventions improved subjects' knowledge about epilepsy. For example, the authors conducted the "Epi-school" program in Japan, which yielded notable outcomes [20]. Furthermore, other programs, such as MOSES [23], The Seizures and Epilepsy Education (SEE) Program [24, 25], FLIP & FLAP [26], Be Seizure Smart [27], Children's (Epilepsy Program [28]), ACINDES [29], and A psychosocial self-management program for epilepsy [30], among others, have also showcased commendable effectiveness in this regard. The PEPE [31] and Ogata's program in Japan [32] showed significant improvement in knowledge based on subjects' subjective ratings. The FAMOSES [33, 34] program for young PWE is being implemented in Germany. It is a psychosocial educational program for children with epilepsy and their families. It is imperative to teach PWE of young origin to know about epilepsy with a view to the future in order to support epilepsy treatment throughout their lives.

The authors implemented a program named "Epi-school," which targeted individuals diagnosed with epilepsy (PWE) aged 16 years and older and their supporters within the outpatient psychiatry department of a university hospital. The program dealt with the epidemiology and fundamental knowledge of epilepsy, diagnosis and treatment of epilepsy, self-control and prognosis of epilepsy, and psychosocial aspects. The program was managed by two fixed trainers (an epilepsy specialist and a psychiatric nurse specialist) and a multidisciplinary team, including a pharmacist, a psychologist, and a mental health worker, depending on the content of each session. In addition to significant increases in knowledge about epilepsy for patients and relatives before and after the program, positive changes were observed in overall life satisfaction and psychological acceptance of epilepsy as an optimistic illness. In addition to enhancing disease-related knowledge and coping mechanisms, numerous participants also expressed observations regarding alterations in the psychological aspects of the disease. Further research is warranted to examine the changes in the self-stigmatization levels of PWE before and after the psychosocial education program.

3.3.2 Psychological support

Epileptic seizures may cause emotional distress and social isolation in PWE. Psychological support is essential to reduce self-stigma, and psychotherapy and counseling, in particular, may promote patients' mental health and reduce self-stigma. Psychological support includes counseling, acceptance and commitment therapy (ACT) [35, 36], cognitive behavioral therapy (CBT), relaxation methods, mindfulness, and motivational interviewing. Some psychosocial education programs mentioned in the previous section also offer psychosocial and psychological support.

Psychological support may be provided within psychosocial education programs, but individual psychotherapy and psychotherapy may benefit PWE who experience self-stigma, even in settings where dedicated psychosocial programs are unavailable.

3.3.3 Support groups, self-help groups

Support and self-help groups are places where people with the same illness can share information and experiences. For PWE, support and self-help groups can reduce feelings of isolation and anxiety by letting them know that others are going through similar experiences. Patients can increase their self-acceptance and reduce self-stigma by participating in support groups. In the context of self-help groups dedicated to epilepsy worldwide, enormous organizations have been established in various countries, including notable examples such as the Japan Epilepsy Association [37], the Epilepsy Foundation [38] in the United States, Epilepsy Action [39] in the United Kingdom, and Epilepsy Action Australia [40] in Australia. These organizations offer a range of information, consultation services and support activities pertaining to epilepsy. However, it is worth noting that the number of organizations operating on a global scale remains limited.

From the authors' survey, in Japan, the use of psychosocial support, that is, participating in epilepsy self-help groups and educational programs, was 5.8% [41]. As a reason for not participating in self-help groups, PWE in Japan worry that they might be discriminated against by society for participating in such groups. In order to effectively address and mitigate self-stigmatization experienced by PWE throughout their lifespans, it is vital to create an environment where PWE feel at ease engaging in self-help groups and study groups. Thus, constant efforts must be directed toward reducing the societal stigma associated with epilepsy and preventing the emergence of new self-stigmatizing beliefs among PWE.

4. Conclusion

This paper introduces the present situation regarding the stigma of epilepsy in Japan and attempts to reduce it, inspired by the authors' research findings. Healthcare professionals involved in epilepsy care must take positive action to prevent the continuation of inadequate knowledge, superstition, and prejudice. Research on self-stigmatization in relation to epilepsy remains limited, underscoring the necessity to develop assessment tools and intervention strategies informed by cross-national findings while accounting for cultural nuances and the specific circumstances surrounding the management of epilepsy in individual countries.

It is imperative to acknowledge that Goffman, the pioneer of the stigma concept, emphasized the significance of understanding stigma as a "relationship" rather than a mere attribute of an individual. This perspective holds spectacular importance in epilepsy, as it is insufficient to perceive epilepsy stigma solely as a characteristic of the individual with epilepsy. Consistent with Goffman's original proposition, it is crucial to conduct research that delves into the process of stigma formation within the psychosocial context of interactions between individuals with epilepsy and their immediate environment and the broader society.

We hope that developing the Epilepsy Self-Stigma Scale (ESSS) and psychosocial education programs presented here will assist this effort and further expand research activities to reduce self-stigma in PWE.

Acknowledgements

We appreciate Dr. Lester Luo's invaluable assistance in editing this manuscript in English.

Funding

This work was supported by the 31st Ochiai Memorial Award Research Grant (2020) and JSPS KAKENHI (No. 21 K13709) and the Maruki Memorial Special Award Research Grant (2022, No.22-1A-01). The funding source was not involved in the design of this study, the writing of this report, and the decision to submit the manuscript for publication.

Declaration of competing interests

None.

Author details

Izumi Kuramochi[1*], Takayuki Iwayama[1,2] and Sakie Shimotsu[3]

1 Department of Psychiatry, Saitama Medical Center, Saitama Medical University, Japan

2 Department of Psychology, Showa Women's University, Japan

3 Faculty of Human Development and Education, Kyoto Women's University, Japan

*Address all correspondence to: kizumi@saitama-med.ac.jp

References

[1] Corrigan PW, Rao D. On the self-stigma of mental illness: Stages, disclosure, and strategies for change. Canadian Journal of Psychiatry. 2012;**57**(8):464-469. DOI: 10.1177/070674371205700804

[2] Kuramochi I, Iwayama T, Oga K, Shiganami T, Umemura T, Kobayashi S, et al. Internet survey on knowledge and perceptions of epilepsy among the general publicinJapan.Heliyon.2022;**8**(12):e12254. DOI: 10.1016/j.heliyon.2022.e12254 eCollection 2022 Dec

[3] Goffman E. Stigma: Notes on the Management of Spoiled Identity. New York: Simon & Schuster; 1963

[4] Jacoby A, Snape D, Baker GA. Epilepsy and social identity: The stigma of a chronic neurological disorder. Lancet Neurology. 2005;**4**:171-178

[5] Baker GA. The psychosocial burden of epilepsy. Epilepsia. 2002;**43**:26-30

[6] Jacoby A. Epilepsy and the quality of everyday life. Findings from a study of people with well-controlled epilepsy. Social Science & Medicine. 1992;**34**:657-666

[7] Mclin WM, de Boer HM. Public perceptions about epilepsy. Epilepsia. 1995;**36**:957-959

[8] Morrel MJ. Stigma and epilepsy. Epilepsy & Behavior. 2002;**3**:21-25

[9] Watson AC, Corrigan PW, Larson JE, Sells M. Self-stigma in people with mental illness. Schizophrenia Bulletin. 2007;**33**:1312-1318

[10] Sirey JA, Bruce ML, Alexopoulos GS, et al. Stigma as a barrier to recovery: Perceived stigma and patient-rated severity of illness as predictors of antidepressant drug adherence. Psychiatric Services. 2001;**52**(12):1615-1620

[11] Sirey JA, Bruce ML, Alexopoulos GS, et al. Perceived stigma as a predictor of treatment discontinuation in young and older outpatients with depression. American Journal of Psychiatry. 2001;**158**(3):479-481

[12] Link B. Understanding labeling effects in the area of mental disorders: An assessment of the effects of expectations of rejection. American Sociological Review. 1987;**52**:96-112

[13] Link B, Cullen F, Struening E, et al. A modified labeling theory approach to mental disorders: An empirical assessment. American Sociological Review. 1989;**54**(3):400-423

[14] Corrigan PW, Watson A, Barr L. The self-stigma of mental illness: Implications for self-esteem and self-efficacy. Journal of Social & Clinical Psychology. 2006;**25**(9):875-884

[15] World Health Organization (WHO). Epilepsy: A public health imperative. 2019. Available from: https://www.who.int/publications/i/item/epilepsy-a-public-health-imperative [accessed 2021-11-30]

[16] Reis R, Meinardi H. ILAE/WHO "Out of the Shadows Campaign" Stigma: Does the flag identify the cargo? Epilepsy & Behavior. 2002;**3**(6S2):33-37

[17] World Health Organization (WHO). Intersectoral global action plan on epilepsy and other neurological disorders 2022-2031. Available

from: https://www.who.int/news/item/28-04-2022-draft-intersectoral-global-action-plan-on-epilepsy-and-other-neurological-disorders-2022-2031 [accessed 2022-11-3]

[18] World Health Organization (WHO). Improving the lives of people with epilepsy –technical brief. 2022. Available from: https://www.who.int/news/item/12-12-2022-new-who-brief-sets-out-actions-needed-to-improve-lives-of-people-with-epilepsyt/news/item/12-12-2022-new-who-brief-sets-out actions-needed-to-improve-lives-of-people-with-epilepsy

[19] Kuramochi I, Horikawa N, Shimotsu S, et al. The self-stigma of patients with epilepsy in Japan: A qualitative approach. Epilepsy & Behavior. 2020;**109**:106994

[20] Kuramochi I, Oga K, Iwayama T, et al. Pilot trial of "Epi-school" group psychosocial education program for patients with epilepsy and their relatives in Japan. Epilepsy & Behavior. 2020;**113**:107545

[21] Kuramochi I, Iwayama T, Horikawa N, et al. Development and validation of the epilepsy self-stigma scale. Epilepsia Open. 2021;**6**(4):748-756

[22] Mittan RJ. Psychosocial treatment programs in epilepsy: A review. Epilepsy & Behavior. 2009;**16**(3):371-380

[23] May TW, Pfafflin M. The efficacy of educational treatment program for patients with epilepsy (MOSES): Results of a controlled, randomized study. Epilepsia. 2002;**43**:539-549

[24] Helgeson DC, Mittan R, Tan SY, Chayasirisobhon S. Sepulveda Epilepsy education: the efficacy of a psychoeducational treatment program in treating medical and psychosocial aspects of epilepsy. Epilepsia. 1990;**31**:75-82

[25] Shore CP, Perkins SM, Austin JK. The seizures and epilepsy education (SEE) program for families of children with epilepsy: A preliminary study. Epilepsy & Behavior. 2008;**12**:157-164

[26] Jantzen S, Muller-Godeffroy E, Hallfahrt-Krisl T, et al. FLIP&FLAP: A training programme for children and adolescents with epilepsy, and their parents. Seizure. Sep 2009;**18**(7):478-486. DOI: 10.1016/j.seizure.2009.04.007

[27] Austin JK, McNelis AM, Shore CP, Dunn DW, Musick B. A feasibility study of a family seizure management program: "Be Seizure Smart". Journal of Neuroscience Nursing. 2002;**34**:30-37

[28] Lewis MA, Salas I, de la Sota A, Chiofalo N, Leake B. Randomized trial of a program to enhance the competencies of children with epilepsy. Epilepsia. 1990;**31**:101-109

[29] Tieffenberg JA, Wood EI, Alonso A, Tossutti MS, Vicente MF. A randomized field trial of ACINDES: A child-centered training model for children with chronic illnesses (asthma and epilepsy). Journal of Urban Health. 2000;**77**:280-297

[30] Pramuka M, Hendrickson R, Zinski A, Van Cott AC. A psychosocial self-management program for epilepsy: A randomized pilot study in adults. Epilepsy & Behavior. 2007;**11**(4):533-545

[31] Huber B, Seidel M. PEPE: A psychoeducative programme for people with epilepsy and learning disabilities. In: Pfafflin M, Frasier RT, Specht U, Thorbeck R, editors. Comprehensive Care for People with Epilepsy. France: John Libbey Eurotext; 2001. pp. 155-162

[32] Ogata A, Amano K. A psychosocial approach to epileptic patients. Epilepsia. 2000;**41**(Suppl. 9):36-38

[33] Wohlrab GC, Rinnert S, Bettendorf U, Fischbach H, Heinen G, Klein P, et al. Famoses Project Group. famoses: A modular educational program for children with epilepsy and their parents. Epilepsy & Behavior. 2007;**10**(1):44-48. DOI: 10.1016/j.yebeh.2006.10.005 Epub 2006 Nov 27

[34] Hagemann A, Pfäfflin M, Nussbeck FW, May TW. The efficacy of an educational program for parents of children with epilepsy (FAMOSES): Results of a controlled multicenter evaluation study. Epilepsy & Behavior. 2016;**64**(Pt A):143-151. DOI: 10.1016/j.yebeh.2016.09.027 Epub 2016 Oct 13

[35] Lundgren T, Dahl J, Yardi N, Melin L. Commitment therapy and yoga for drug-refractory epilepsy: A randomized controlled trial. Epilepsy & Behavior. 2008;**13**:102-108

[36] Lundgren T, Dahl J, Melin L, Kies B. Evaluation of acceptance and commitment therapy for drug refractory epilepsy: A randomized controlled trial in South Africa—a pilot study. Epilepsia. 2006;**47**:2173-2179

[37] The Japan Epilepsy Association. Available from: https://jes-jp.org/en/ [accessed 2023-5-17]

[38] The Epilepsy Foundation. Available from: https://www.jea-net.jp/ [accessed 2023-5-17]

[39] Epilepsy Action. Available from: https://www.epilepsy.com/ [accessed 2023-5-17]

[40] Epilepsy Action Australia. Available from: https://www.epilepsy.org.au/ [accessed 2023-5-17]

[41] Kuramochi I, Iwayama T, Oga K, Shiganami T, Umemura T, Kobayashi S, et al. A study of factors influencing self-stigma in people with epilepsy: A nationwide online questionnaire survey in Japan. Epilepsia Open. 2022;**7**(4):792-801. DOI: 10.1002/epi4.12661 Epub 2022 Oct 25